I0521002

INTERSECTION

OF PAIN, HOPE,

AND FAITH

None of us are born knowing how to overcome physical
and emotional pain on our own. We all need help from someone
who cares for our well-being.

INTERSECTION

OF PAIN, HOPE,

AND FAITH

A Confrontation
Between the Mind, Body, and Soul

Paula Phillips

Copyrighted Material

Intersection of Pain, Hope, and Faith
A Confrontation Between the Mind, Body, and Soul

Copyright © 2025 by Calibrating Lyfe Publishing. All Rights Reserved.

No part of this publication may be reproduced, stored in a retrieval
system or transmitted, in any form or by any means—electronic, mechanical,
photocopying, recording or otherwise—without prior written permission from
the publisher, except for the inclusion of brief quotations in a review.

For information about this title or to order other books
and/or electronic media, contact the publisher:

Calibrating Lyfe Publishing
http://calibratinglyfe.com
info@calibratinglyfe.com

ISBNs:
979-8-9985890-1-0 (hardcover)
979-8-9985890-0-3 (softcover)
979-8-9985890-2-7 (eBook)

Printed in the United States of America

Cover and Interior design: 1106 Design

Disclaimer

This book provides information regarding the subject matter covered.
It is sold with the understanding that the publisher and the author are
not engaged in rendering psychological or medical advice.

The sample patient references are based on a collection of several common medical conditions
that are treated in the healthcare field. They are used for illustrative purposes only.

Dedication

First, I dedicate this book to my Lord and Savior, Jesus Christ. Without His grace, I would not be able to share this universal story of the struggle with physical, psychological, and spiritual pain and strategies to overcome them. Second, I dedicate this book to my phenomenal husband. You never backed down from the dark days and long nights. Thank you for your unconditional love and support.

Letter to Reader

Dear Reader,

My purpose for writing to you is to impart all that I have gleaned from my encounter with severe physical pain in the hope that my testimony and the observations I've made will be of use for other teetering souls in the fight of their life against the enemies within: chronic pain, depression, and doubt. I hope my personal experience and professional insight can help someone avoid the almost inevitable road to desolation when navigating the pitfalls of severe pain.

May courage and hope abide in you,

Paula Phillips

Contents

Introduction

According to the 2020 census, of the 331,449.28 million people in the United States over 100 million meet the criteria for chronic pain syndrome and disabling chronic pain. That means that one-third of the population is physically suffering with pain, along with the daily stressors of living, and many are besieged with the emotional toll of the pain disease.[1,2]

Chronic pain, be it back pain, migraine, or joint pain, can profoundly disrupt a person's life, leading to career loss, depression, anxiety—even poverty. Studies show that persons with chronic pain face a higher risk of mental health issues, due to the sudden traumatic changes which can lead to disability. Every area of a person's life is affected by debilitating pain, a multifaceted disease that is not confined to a single body part.[3,4]

Unfortunately, chronic pain has a much greater impact on society than the top three chronic long-term diseases: diabetes, high blood pressure, and cancer.[5] Currently, 52.4 people out of 1,000 are newly diagnosed with chronic pain each year. This outpaces the number of high blood pressure diagnoses (45.3 out of a sample of 1,000), and diabetes diagnoses (7.1 out of 1,000).[6] This makes chronic pain the most common long-term disease people face.

Each individual's introduction into the chronic pain community varies, but the landscape of days lived with a disability is universal, and the emotional and financial toll of chronic pain is a global problem. The Global Burden of Disease, an independent population health research organization, reported that "the high prominence of pain, and diseases associated with pain, as a global cause of disability in both developed and developing countries, with chronic low back pain as the single greatest cause of disability internationally.[7,8]

In the U.S., the annual direct medical costs and lost wages associated with pain disability are higher than the combined cost and wage losses for cancer, heart disease, and diabetes combined.[9,10] This implies that beyond the burden of disability, the financial burden of chronic pain is greater than the two leading causes of death: heart disease and cancer.[11]

Due to the innumerable aspects of pain and the permanent changes it causes over time in the nervous system and the brain, chronic pain is now viewed globally more as a disease—not just a symptom. Regarding pain as a disease means medical professionals can consider a more comprehensive intervention approach. I believe this distinction opens the door for a more wholistic view of the condition, one that considers the impact of pain on mental health.

The symbiotic relationship between chronic pain and mental illness is apparent in the high percentage of individuals who become depressed or whose existing depression escalates with the onset of chronic pain. Although chronic pain is an accelerant to several mental illnesses and undermines a person's response to pain management interventions, chronic pain is still treated by some in the medical field as an isolated symptom.

Medical professionals who view the onset of chronic pain as a mere symptom prioritize the physical pain and neglect to address the psychological pain that research shows intensifies the pain experience.[12] Unfortunately, a person in this scenario becomes vulnerable to the compounding effects of emotional and physical disability, and their mental health suffers. Should the global medical community abandon this tunnel-vision approach to chronic pain, it would create an early opportunity to more inclusively account for the multitude of emotional and psychosocial variables that complicate recovery.

As an occupational therapist and a physical rehabilitation practitioner, I've seen the negative impact of chronic pain and depression on an individual's ability to recover from illnesses and injuries. Their recovery is typically much slower, or stalls out compared to the recovery of a person without chronic pain and depression diagnoses.

I specialize in identifying the minute parts of the whole-body system that enables a person to physically, emotionally, and cognitively function. The human body is a conglomeration of intricate systems orchestrated to sustain life. It is composed of the following systems: circulatory (heart), digestive (eating and digesting food), endocrine (hormones), immune (cells, organs, molecules), integumentary (skin), renal (kidneys), respiratory (breathing), musculoskeletal (muscles and bones), nervous (brain and nerves), and the reproductive system. The final system—the psychosocial system—is not technically or medically included in the body systems as it is not an anatomical or physical structure. It is, however, essential to how we engage in life and encompasses mental health and the social influences that impact an individual's well-being.

My expertise is in using rehabilitative methods to mitigate the malfunctioning aspects in the physiological and psychological systems that prevent a person from being able to do the things they need and want to do in everyday life. I apply therapeutic frameworks and techniques to address physical and mental health issues that hinder daily functioning.

Take a person with chronic pain, depression, and anxiety who has sustained a head or spinal injury from a car accident. If they can no longer feed themselves, one of their recovery goals will be to regain this ability. To help them accomplish that, I must determine the following: Which muscle groups and sensory systems enable them to reach for a fork, pierce their food, and bring it to their mouth; which area of the brain controls these muscle groups; and which brain area enables them to identify silver objects as a fork and knife, a round porcelain object as a plate, and items on the plate as food.

Sadly, due to any preexisting mental health issues, they may perceive the accident as yet another disabling, uncontrollable life event, develop feelings of overwhelming helplessness, and disengage from contributing to their quality of life. They also tend to no longer value the need to care for themselves. My role is to develop and implement a treatment plan that encompasses physical and mental health strategies to facilitate their active engagement in their recovery.

During my own experience with injury and severe pain, my professional understanding of the complex aspects of recovery was rendered useless. I'd thought that being a healthcare professional, an empathetic scientist accustomed to the methodology of healing, recovery, and pain, gave me an advantage that would prepare me to deal with my sudden back injury. In fact, in the early stages of my injury, my confidence soared due to my knowledge about the rehabilitative process. My doctor also indicated a favorable outcome for recovery because I exercised, had a healthy lifestyle, and ate a nutritious, well-balanced diet.

But as my pain lingered, I realized how much I'd prided myself on my professional acumen, which now felt as useless as a wool coat in the Sahara Desert. My so-called education and training did not prepare me for what I would personally experience. I didn't anticipate what lay dormant in my body and mind, waiting for an opportune time to emerge.

Introduction

To my surprise, the relentless, torturous nature of the physical and psychological pain from my injury undermined my intellect and experience. Severe pain is a ravenous enemy within that consumes everything in its path, destroying the fabric of human life while unraveling the tapestry of faith.

With depression to my right and severe pain to my left, I was trapped between two enemies within. The fragile walls of my mind confined me in a dark, cold, lonely place. My North Star of faith dimmed. I stumbled, falling into an abyss of failed hope, and my vanquished soul plummeted into despondency.

Pain became a mirror that reflected the hubris in my personal, professional, and spiritual life. It was impossible to look away from the image of despair staring back at me. Desperate for a path to healing, I eventually realized there was a missing ingredient in the prescription for healing my doctors and pharmacist could not fill.

My personal experience compelled me to scrutinize the intersectionality of faith, hope, and physical pain—key parts of our well-being to have a fulfilled life with chronic pain. Understanding these factors at a granular level can enable chronic pain sufferers to overcome the devastation inherent in debilitating pain and disability.

I believe knowing the function and the process of faith, hope, and pain is essential for individuals to avoid the coercive force of chronic pain and to develop vital coping strategies for living well.

CHAPTER ONE

Injured

to be physically hurt; to be impaired;
to be damaged; to be broken

My patients and their families often ask what motivated me to undertake the unglamorous work of teaching people how to care for themselves and manage their lives after an injury or an illness. Why did I choose to help those unable, and at times unwilling, to help themselves? Why did I choose to use my body as lever and external stabilizer to move their debilitated or paralyzed arms and legs into a functional position?

My response has always been: I am the lucky one. I can help others whose lives are disrupted by illness, injury, an elective surgery gone wrong—or a surgery that goes right and requires only instruction to modify their daily activities during the recovery process. I tell them my career is a calling. I am privileged to harness my expertise and compassion to improve the quality of life for those needing to navigate their "new" life.

~

It was a typical day at work. The first of the nine patients I helped had their life upended by a severe stroke—not one that causes total disability, but close. I've seen my share of those, and it's profoundly heartbreaking. My emotions are stirred every time I meet my patients—first on paper, when I read their often-tragic medical history. Then, I meet them in person when I walk into their hospital room and greet them while they are lying in a bed.

"Hello. My name is Paula, and I'll be your Occupational Therapist. I understand you've had a stroke. Strokes disrupt the nervous system signals from your brain to your body and from your body to your brain. Your brain is the control center for your body and nervous system. Those systems send and receive instructions through your thoughts to control how your body moves. The nervous system also sends and receives automatic instructions from within your body, which does not require your thoughts to control what your body does. For example, we don't have to think about breathing; our body automatically breathes.

"The stroke injured the left side of your brain, causing weakness on the right side of your body. This is called hemiparesis, or a muscular weakness to one side of the body. The stroke also caused you to have difficulty organizing your thoughts and finding the words you want to say. This is called aphasia.

"It's also difficult to straighten your arm. This condition is called muscular spasticity. This happens because the stroke injures the brain causing damage to the pathway and the signal that allows your arm muscles to relax (straighten) and contract (bend). The malfunctioning signal from your nervous system causes your arm to spontaneously bend at the elbow. When you try to straighten your arm and reach for your eyeglasses on the table, the muscles in your bicep tighten and become rigid. This makes it impossible for you to extend your arm in front of you. The faulty signals from your injured nervous system cannot deliver the correct message for your arm to 'reach,' 'stretch forward,' or 'pick up the eyeglasses.'

"Your stroke has also made it difficult for you to see things on the right side of your field of vision. Although your eyesight is normal, the stroke injured the part of the brain that controls visual attention and awareness. 'Visual attention' is the ability to focus on a task, person, or object within your field of vision. You are also not aware of the right side of your body and objects positioned on your right side. This is called visual hemispatial neglect. When your visual awareness is impaired, you do not internally or automatically perceive anything in your right visual field.

"The stroke has made it difficult for you to do many basic things, such as sitting up on the edge of the bed, standing, walking, and controlling urination and bowel movements.

"My job is to help you recover and retrain your brain, nervous system, and muscular system so you can once again do routine daily living tasks such as dressing and bathing, managing your hygiene, getting in and out of the shower and bed, and getting on and off a commode. I will also address how your stroke has affected your ability to continue to engage in other essential aspects of your life: your hobbies, your work, and intimacy with your partner.

"The medical community calls these areas Activities of Daily Living (ADLs) and Instrumental Activities of Daily Living (IADL). My purpose is to enable you to have the best quality of life and the highest level of performance and independence. I will teach you and your family strategies to overcome the physical and neuromuscular impairments that have the greatest impact on your functional abilities. These impairments can be slow to recover when an injury to the brain occurs, but I will also teach you how to adapt to these sudden changes that have disrupted your daily routine and lifestyle

"I know all this is overwhelming, and I understand your embarrassment and frustration. Having this type of injury to your nervous system and depending on someone else to do basic things for you is an extremely uncomfortable and vulnerable place to be in. You may feel you've been stripped of the control of your life. But please know that I am here to help you reach your goal to regain self-sufficiency in the areas the stroke has impacted.

"Your condition is very common, and I have many years of experience and a lot of training that will be useful for you. I will use many therapeutic processes to help your brain develop new neurological pathways to communicate with your body. In addition, I will also use several therapeutic techniques for your nervous system to once again send normal signals to your body. This can be a long and arduous process but improvement is possible.

"Let's start by you allowing me to guide your body from lying on your back to sitting on the right side of your bed. I know you cannot move your right arm and leg, but every time I give you instructions for the right side of your body, I want you to think about doing what I am asking, and I will move your arm and leg for you. Thinking about what you want the right side of your body to do and attempting to move starts the recovery process. I will instruct you slowly as I physically guide you through every step. This is beginning the process of retraining the body to function and respond correctly.

"I know you don't have the balance to sit up alone because you fall over to the right, toward your weak side. I'll be supporting you completely by standing directly in front of you and stabilizing you with both my hands, one on each of your shoulders. My legs will straddle around yours. The inside of my knees will be against the outside of your knees so I can stabilize your right leg. I'll demonstrate this with your wife so you can see what I mean.

"Now it's time to sit up on the edge of the bed. First, bend your left knee. Now, bend your right knee. Move your right arm slightly toward the edge of the bed, away from your body, so it doesn't get pinned when you roll over to your right side. Now push both of your heels into the mattress and try to slightly lift your bottom up away from the mattress and scoot your hips over to the left. Now with your left arm, reach for the bed rail on the right side of the bed. Now roll onto your right side and move your legs off the bed. I am going to lean over you and put my hands around your shoulders. When you feel me pulling you upright, I want you to push yourself up with your left arm at the same time.

"I know you're nervous, but don't push against me; that will make it difficult for me to physically help you. I promise I won't let you fall off the bed; I won't let go of you. It may be difficult now, but it will get easier.

"Now that you're sitting, please place both hands on the bed beside you to stabilize yourself. I will help you straighten your right arm. It's a positive sign that I could place your hand on the bed; it means the spasticity in your right arm is not too rigid. You're doing very well for someone who hasn't been out of bed in five weeks. Now that you're sitting, please turn your head to the left and then to the right until you see your wife smiling at you. That was a good attempt. Now please place your left hand on top of your right hand. I know it's difficult, because you must turn your head to find your right hand.

"We'll continue to work on your visual tracking, your overall strength, your arm function, and your balance. You've been sitting for fifteen minutes—that's quite an accomplishment. Now I'll help you lie back down on the bed. Thank you for trusting me. I will do the best I can to help you reach your goals."

Now it was time to develop and implement the most effective treatment plan for the remaining patients on my schedule to rehabilitate their musculoskeletal, cognitive, nervous, and visual motor systems. To devise the most effective plan, I consider the full scope of the physical and emotional changes that occur when an individual's health issues upend their life. It's imperative that I address their psychological needs—anxiety, stress, fear, depression, coping behavior—and their psychosocial needs, including how their culture, family, and societal views impact their self-image and well-being.

$$\sim$$

I said adiós to the end of a nonstop week, as I walked to my car. The parking lot was surrounded by trees with amber leaves announcing autumn's arrival. The crisp fresh fall scented breeze made me ready for a cozy Friday night around the fire.

The next morning, the sun was peeping through the blinds, but I was not ready to leave my comfy bed. Instead, I planned a full day of errands from the warm embrace of my cozy velvety blanket.

I convinced myself I needed a quick twenty-minute jog on the treadmill followed by some light weightlifting since I'd skipped my 8:00 a.m. Pilates class and planned to indulge in brunch at our favorite restaurant. My husband and I would have our usual toast with cranberry mimosas.

I would have a side of eggs, fresh fruit, and the harvest pecan pancakes that always had the right amount of cinnamon, whipped butter, and warm maple syrup. After that, my husband would transform from my Saturday morning date to our teenage son's personal Uber driver and I'd become his chatty front-seat passenger. Around sunset, nestled in my favorite sweats, I'd sit on the patio sipping on a pumpkin spice latte until the chilly evening ushered us indoors. But first, I had to get my lazy bones out of bed.

In typical fashion, I rolled over to sit up—and a sudden cramping pressure in my lower back made it difficult to get up. I thought I must have strained a muscle at work because it was unusual for me to have a backache.

I replayed my hectic week of helping patients of all levels of physical dependence, focusing on those who required the most physical assistance. That's because a back strain is typically caused by incorrect body mechanics when helping someone stand or lift their arms/legs, or lifting someone I'm not strong enough to assist on my own. I'd helped a few patients who'd placed me at the highest risk of injuring my back.

I concentrated on Thursday and Friday, because the onset of pain is usually 24 to 48 hours from the time of injury.

There was the 6'3" patient who weighed around 340 pounds and was too weak to sit on the side of the bed or to stand. Three other people helped me roll him from lying on his back onto his side because he didn't have enough upper body strength to use the rails on the hospital bed to move himself in the bed. Since he was also unable to sit stand, I used a mechanical lift designed to transfer people out of bed into a wheelchair.

Another patient was five inches taller and a weighed 100 pounds more than me, at 5'10" and 240 pounds. I'd taught them how to maintain their balance while standing and to pivot from the wheelchair using a grab bar on the wall beside the commode for support. I needed to use about half of my strength to help fulfill that patient's most important goal—being able to use the restroom instead of an adult diaper or bed pan.

The last potential patient I could have strained my back assisting was 5'8" and 195 pounds. He had an amputated right leg and a right shoulder injury. I taught this individual to use a transfer board (Figure A) to get in and out of the bed and onto a drop arm bedside commode (Figure B). A transfer/sliding board is a 24-inch wooden board used as a bridge from a bed, chair, or commode. It is used for mobilizing patients to those surfaces when they are unable to stand.

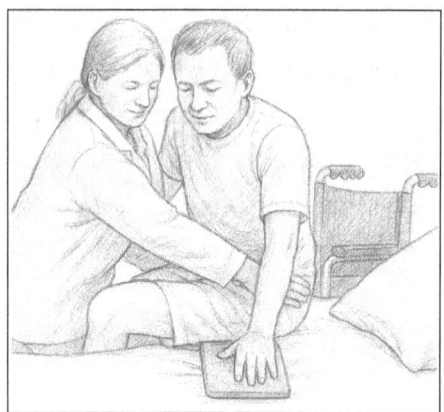

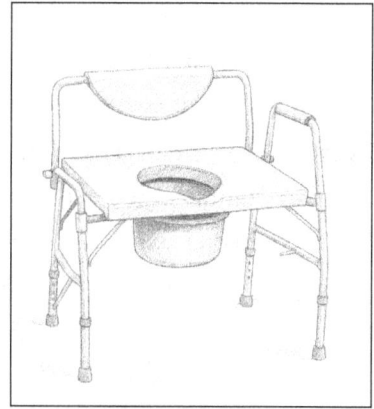

Figure A: Transfer/Sliding Board

Figure B: Drop Arm Bedside Commode

Scrutinizing my body mechanics from the previous week provided no reasonable explanation for the nagging cramp in my lower back. And since I'd done nothing out of the ordinary at home, I couldn't find a reasonable explanation for my pain. I jokingly asked my husband, "Did you hear me fall out of the bed last night?"

Laughing, he said, "You slept in an awkward position—on your stomach. When I tried to get you to turn over to your back you kept moving to your side and then back on your stomach."

Ordinarily that would not be a strange position. But we have an adjustable-base bedframe, with the head and foot sections elevated in "zero gravity." Both are slightly raised, with the foot of the bed slightly higher. The intended sleep position is on one's back. But I'd slept on my stomach, in a position similar to a yoga "Superman" pose, for an unknown amount of time throughout the night (Figure C). This position is not ideal, because the lower spine is bent in the area where it should be straight.

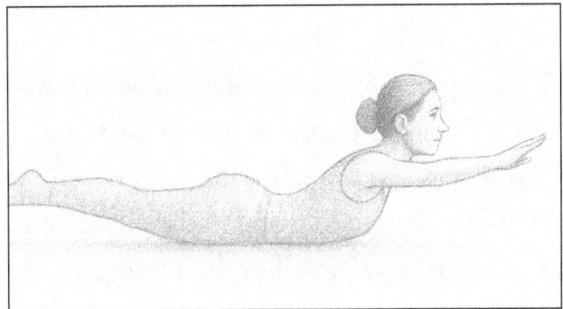

Figure C

After hearing my husband's eyewitness report, I concluded that my lower back muscles were strained from being in an awkward position. After an hour of piddling around the house, waiting for the Motrin to take effect, spasms began to pommel my lower back and thighs.

Brunch was cancelled and our weekend plans now included binge-watching Netflix, watching college football, and reading. The snack menu would include chilled lime-flavored Topo Chico sparkling water, popcorn, warm chocolate chip cookies, and hot green tea for its anti-inflammatory benefits. I also initiated a protocol like-minded healthcare professionals would recommend for treating a muscle strain: Apply ice to the injured area, rest that area, and alternate Motrin and Tylenol for the next few days. I was certain this muscle strain would be resolved by the end of the week at most.

~

Back Sprain—Day 1

"Hi, I'm Paula, and I'll be your occupational therapist today. I understand that you've been in the hospital for over two months because of complications from COVID-19. I'd like to discuss your medical history and your prior level of function before you had COVID and the treatment plan I'll develop to help you get back on your feet and get home. Before your COVID diagnoses, you were working full-time, minimally exercising, and able to go up and down the stairs in your home, shop in stores, drive, take care of yourself, stand in the shower to bathe yourself without help from your spouse, walk without using a cane, and had no history of falls at home.

"Your only pre-existing medical condition was high blood pressure and depression. However, since having COVID you've developed diabetes, heart failure, dizziness, muscular weakness all over your body, an unexplained inability to balance yourself when sitting and standing, a difficult time remembering things, difficulty concentrating, and respiratory failure that has resulted in your dependence on supplemental oxygen to breathe comfortably. As a result, you're no longer able to take care of yourself and do what you were physically and mentally able to normally do.

"I'm truly sorry this has happened, and I can imagine how this is affecting you and your family. After assessing your strength, standing and sitting balance, coordination, cognition, and your respiratory system's ability to meet the oxygen demands of your body, I've developed an occupational therapy plan of care to help you recover."

After leaving that patient's room, I had to be mindful of *my* plan of care for my back recovery. For the next few days, I refrained from physically overextending myself at work. I did not help anyone stand or get out of bed into a wheelchair if they required a significant amount of assistance from me. I took Motrin to reduce the inflammation in my lower back muscles and decreased the amount of time I spent standing at work and at home. It was common for me to stand for three hours at a time at home if I was busy cleaning the house and meal prepping for the week. In addition, I put my routine exercise regimen of using the elliptical, running, and weight training on hold.

I removed inflammatory foods such as dairy, gluten, tomatoes, red meat, fried and processed foods, and lessened my sugar intake to decrease the overall inflammation in my body. In the beginning, I didn't consider my symptoms to be too much of a problem because I have a high tolerance for pain. My low back strain and frequent spasms were merely an inconvenience. I just needed to make minor adjustments to avoid aggravating my already irritated muscles.

Day 5

I had a typical schedule of patients: ten people I needed to help reach the best possible outcome for their medical conditions. Because my symptoms were not subsiding, I was more cautious than usual with my hands-on facilitative therapeutic methods that required me to lift patients' arms and legs. I began to scrutinize their diagnosis, height, and weight, to determine if I was physically capable of providing occupational therapy services.

The adjustments I made were becoming more obvious to my observant colleagues, who recognized something was wrong. Lightheartedly, I explained I'd strained a muscle in my back. But the back strain was not improving. In fact, it was getting worse.

It was becoming too uncomfortable to sit at my desk to complete the documentation in the patients' medical records. I changed my desk chair and brought a specialty pillow from home. This allowed me to sit with less discomfort.

I treated myself as an outpatient therapy client with a diagnosis of back strain to improve the time frame for recovery. During lunch breaks, I alternated using all of our rehabilitation department's therapeutic modalities. I used transcutaneous electrical nerve stimulation (TENS), a device that delivers an electric current through the skin that activates nerve fibers to reduce pain. I also used Shortwave Diathermy, a device that uses electromagnetic current in the form of radio waves or micro-waves to reduce pain and inflammation. Depending on my symptoms, I also applied an icepack any time I sat for longer than twenty minutes.

During this time, the pain from my spine to the back of my knees felt like a million needle pokes per minute that caused a frequent, sporadic electric shock sensation. The persistent spasms in my legs and back mocked my first line of offense: rest, modalities, ibuprofen, and Tylenol. Dreading the thought of another achy weekend, I made an appointment with my doctor.

Again, armed with years of expertise, I wasn't surprised by my physician's recommendation: a five-day dose pack of steroids to decrease inflammation and a muscle relaxer to reduce spasms. The prescribed medications did not disappoint; this second-line of offense put me even closer to recovery. I also implemented these adaptations to support the healing process: I adjusted my work schedule to permit sitting more often and I treated fewer patients to shorten my workday.

Relying on the additional benefit of over-the-counter pain relievers and the therapeutic modalities I treated myself with at work, I was able to continue my physically demanding job. I was on the one-yard line to defeat this muscle strain and better able to manage my workday, where sitting for more than two hours is a rare luxury and constant standing, bending, walking, lifting patients' arms, legs, and bodies when they cannot move them themselves is standard as a member of an inpatient rehabilitation team. However, the saying, "all good things come to an end," could not be truer.

Day 10

As Cinderella had experienced, at the stroke of midnight the elation of better days began to disappear. I expected the back strain to be fully resolved once the steroid prescription ended. But day by day, I was becoming more dependent on the maximum dosage of the over-the-counter pain medications. It was beginning to feel like I was taking a placebo instead of the real acetaminophen and ibuprofen.

As my back worsened, the assuredness I'd initially felt deflated my confidence like air from a punctured balloon. The tables turned. I was indeed a patient, my patient, using all the Activities of Daily Living strategies I taught those recovering from a spinal injury or spinal surgery.

I had to adapt how I dressed, slept, bathed, sat, stood, walked, performed my job, and fulfilled my duties at home. I absolutely had to avoid bending, lifting, and twisting. I had to use a 'Reacher', a common piece of adaptive equipment to grasp items that require bending to retrieve.

The intrusion of this "muscle strain" was like a virus hacking my life. I was malfunctioning. Everything I could once do without conscious thought was becoming increasingly difficult—almost impossible. The modifications I made at work morphed into "light duty," the term for being able to work with restricted job duties to prevent exacerbating an injury or medical condition. I was hands-off, only supervising the occupational therapy services provided by assistants.

My quality of life had shifted at the command of this so-called muscle strain. Pain set boundaries for how I did the things I needed and wanted to do. I could not pick my shoes off the floor, put on socks, shave my legs, lean over the sink to wash my face, or casually sit on a chair without volts of what felt like electricity crippling my efforts. I could not lift the blender to make fruit smoothies, unload my dishwasher, or retrieve a plate from the cabinet. I could not carry a bag of groceries, clean my shower, vacuum, or mop the floor. I'm not to saying I was eager to do those chores, but I took for granted that I could. My fall vegetable gardening plans were also postponed.

I altered how I slept—if I could sleep at all—a pillow here, a pillow there, a pillow everywhere: under my arms, my legs, or my head. But there never seemed enough pillows to soften the blows from the spasms that jarred me throughout the night.

Almost every time I took a step, what felt like an electric current running from my lower back to the soles of my feet reminded me of my limits when I walked. Like a well-trained Pavlov dog, to avoid the bolts of electricity, I changed my gait, which no longer resembled normal walking. It was a stiff-legged shuffle. I looked like I was walking with a rope tied around my ankles, constricting every step.

I couldn't make enough modifications to avoid the pain that erupted every time I lowered myself to sit or transitioned to standing. I had to execute sitting and standing with the calculated maneuverability of a gymnast on a balance beam as those transitions became increasingly more impossible.

Day 11

Enough was enough. I needed a different plan. I told my doctor about my worsening symptoms. She thought they were beginning to show telltale signs of spinal nerve complications—not simply muscle strain. She immediately referred me to a renowned neurosurgeon, a specially trained doctor who diagnoses and treats conditions that affect the nerves, brain, spinal cord, and the nervous system. Neurosurgeons perform surgery to correct and repair maladies in the nervous system, but they also provide nonsurgical treatment interventions.

Day 13

During my initial visit, the neurosurgeon completed an assessment that confirmed that a nerve in my lower back was causing my symptoms, not a muscle strain. We discussed short-term use medications to manage the pain. I was adamant about avoiding opioid pain relievers. He acknowledged and respected my concern and did not prescribe any narcotic-based pain relievers. As our conversation continued, he gave me some of the familiar assurances I'd often given to my patients. "You will get through this," he said. "Just take it easy and avoid lifting and doing anything strenuous or anything that causes more pain." Next up on the treatment plan was an appointment for an MRI of the spine. Thankfully, I was able to schedule this for 7:30 p.m. the following day.

Day 15

I finished my day of light duty at work around noon Friday. On my way home, I received a text: the MRI results were in. The undercover muscle strain received its true name: lumbar 4 (L4) and lumbar 5 (L5) bulging lumbar disc.

The lumbar section of the spine, is the waist area, and it comprises five of the spine's thirty-three vertebrae. They are the largest vertebrae in the lower part of the spine, which supports the majority of our weight from the waist up. Bending and rotation are calibrated in the lower back making the lumbar vertebrae the articulating and stability point for the entire spine. It is also the most common source of back pain and injury that causes disability and prevents people from returning to work[13].

Knowing all this, I was not surprised when the neurosurgeon said I could not return to work. I obviously could not meet the physical demands of my job; I was barely meeting the physical demands of my daily life. The extent of my bulging lumbar disc astounded me because typically with an injury this severe I would have done something arduous to cause the injury.

He agreed the sudden presentation of my symptoms was unusual without a definite inciting event. The severity of my bulging disc was attributed to the fact that, as people age, minor disc bulges are common and typically asymptomatic—meaning anyone can have a slightly bulging disc and not know it because they experience no discomfort.

His theory was that I had a preexisting minimal lumbar disc bulge. My work constantly bending, lifting, pushing, pulling, and supporting incapacitated patients had a cumulative impact on this asymptomatic bulging disc. Additionally, sleeping in a prone, extended position put pressure over a prolonged period of time on my compromised lumbar disc. This increased the disc bulge, causing it to worsen and aggravate the surrounding nerve fibers, which were causing my symptoms.

The MRI revealed my disc bulge was serious but not at the point of rupturing. I was concerned, but not afraid. I was relieved to finally know the cause of my pain and that surgery would not be required.

Although debilitating at times, bulging discs are not unusual. The disc, which functions like a cushion or padding between the vertebrae, bulges outside of its usual confined space, touching the nerves situated directly beside the disc. This contact with the nerve causes pain, muscle spasms, and weakness.

We discussed the of leave of absence I'd need to take from work. I'd take short-term disability for four to six weeks because bulging discs take about six to eight weeks to retract to their normal size. The four-to-six-week calculation was based on my injury being two weeks old.

The recommended treatment plan was conservative management. This meant surgery was not part of the plan. Instead, he'd refer me to another doctor, a pain management specialist, to address my symptoms more aggressively.

I'm usually a positive person, one who believes everything will work out—because it always has in my life. Not to say my life was paved with rose petals, but I'd always felt God's presence and grace in my life. So I did what came naturally: focus on the positive, pray, and give the strategy time to work. I thought I had nothing to worry about, because I had a plan of treatment and abundant faith in God.

CHAPTER TWO

Foundation

*the base below the surface
that supports the structure above it*

To better understand where my faith in God originated, I will take you back to my beginnings. The matriarch of our family, my paternal grandmother, was an exceptional woman, and she influenced the trajectory of my spiritual life from a very young age.

She was a regal 5'10" bronze-skinned beauty with dark twinkling eyes, a graceful stride, and a smile that would put a model's smile to shame. Her aura was warm and welcoming—much like a wood-burning fire on a snowy day that draws you near. She had a reassuring embrace that touched the soul and told you everything would be all right. Her wise eyes penetrated beyond the surface of my appearance and often made me wonder: What did she see when she looked so intently at me?

She spoke in a calm, melodic tone saturated with love that embodied the essence of I Corinthians 13:4-6 *New International Version*: "Love is patient, love is kind. It does not envy, it does not boast, it is not proud. It does not dishonor others, it is not self-seeking, it is not easily angered, it keeps no record of wrongs. Love does not delight in evil but rejoices with truth. It always protects, always trusts, always hopes, always perseveres." She never raised her voice and always spoke with patience and compassion.

Her unparalleled affection and wisdom made her a magnet for her grandchildren. She indulged all of us, making each one feel as though we were her favorite. She always had cookies or cake and let us have our fill of the candy bowl. My grandmother had two loves—the Lord Jesus Christ and her family. She told Bible stories in a way that rivaled many of my favorite storybooks. I became enamored with the majestic God she so richly described. She made sure her grandchildren knew God the Father, the Son, and the Holy Spirit.

She told me about God creating all the beautiful things in the world, everything in the sky, the ocean, and the air we breathe. Her voice was filled with enthusiasm and the pitch of her voice went up two octaves when she said, "On top of that, He created you, his most treasured creation. You and all the people in the world are what God loves the most. God is just awesome!" You could feel her love of God and see it in her expression as she spoke about Him.

She explained God's love to me by comparing His love to the way my parents loved me before I was born and how they would do anything to help me, even risk their lives to save me from danger. She said their love would never change or end because I was their child and a part of them. Because my parents loved me so much, they'd always want what was best for me and they'd always want me near them. She explained God loved me the same way. I was His child, a part of him, and He had done everything to save me. And like my parents, He loved me before I was born. God wanted me to be with Him too.

She went on to say that we will live in two places in our lifetime. We will live on Earth for a while to do the "good assignment" God has given us. When we finish our "good work," our life on Earth will end. Then we will live in Heaven, the place where we will be the closest to God. She would say excitedly that the good news is that our life in Heaven will never end; it will be filled with endless days of joy and happiness. She called this eternal life. Loving, believing, and obeying Christ gives us a ticket to get into Heaven, where we will sit with God forever.

Again reminding me of the parallel relationship between my parents and Jesus Christ, she said the expectation and requirement to be respectful, loving, obedient, and honest as well as saying "please" and "thank you" to my parents when I wanted something and received it, and not throw a tantrum when I didn't get what I wanted, was the same requirement and expectation Christ has for me in our relationship. I should be thankful each day and make sure I let the Lord know I love Him. She said the things I do and the words I speak should show that I love God—just like my parents show love toward me every day. The things my parents do for me and the words they say show me they love me and that I am special.

My grandmother always encouraged me to get to know the "Good Lord" because He is a friend when I am lonely or sad. I can talk to Him anytime about anything. When I'm frustrated, confused, or angry, he is there to comfort and calm me. He can give me all I need. She was careful to say this did not include toys on Christmas or my birthday wish list. He is also a protector when I am afraid. Her love and the kindness of Christ compelled me to want to know the "Almighty God," and "Jesus Christ the Son of God," and this "Holy Spirit" she was so found of.

She taught me that baptism was an expression of our commitment to God's instructions for living and believing He is all that He says He is. She would say the commitment we make to God is a sacred promise, an oath that should not be broken. She added that broken promises cause hurt feelings, so it's important to keep promises to each other, especially to God. She shared endless stories and examples of God's love and how Jesus became Christ, always emphasizing that she loved the Lord because He loved us first and we should love Him in return.

Local churches conducted outreach in our inner-city apartment complex where my grandmother and family lived, alongside other middle-class working families. A Baptist church routinely sent a bus to pick up children and others who wished to attend church. On Saturdays, my grandmother would always say, in her sweet Southern voice, "Make sure y'all don't stay up too late and miss the church bus in the morning. It's important for y'all to learn about the Good Lord."

As I child, I don't think I noticed that my parents didn't join us, but they made sure my two older siblings and I attended church regularly. The bus ride to and from church was always fun. We looked forward to eating doughnuts and other snacks the church provided, singing songs, and receiving toys like jacks, yo-yos, and other keepsakes, depending on the season.

One day during Sunday school, God tapped me on the shoulder. The teacher told the story about Moses and the burning bush (Exodus 3:2-10 NIV).* In this scripture, God got Moses's attention with a bush engulfed in flames, yet the leaves and branches were not burning. When Moses inspected the bush to see how this was possible, God called him by name twice. He spoke to Moses about becoming His representative and taking a message to Pharaoh, the king of Egypt.

---

* There the angel of the Lord appeared to him in flames of fire from within a bush. Moses saw that though the bush was on fire it did not burn up. So Moses thought, "I will go over and see this strange site–why the bush does not burn up" . . . God called him from within the bush, "Moses! Moses! . . . I am the God of your father, the God of Abraham. The God of Isaac and the God of Jacob . . . I am sending you to Pharaoh . . .

Like Moses, I was in awe that God could become a flame yet not burn the bush and speak—all at the same time. At the end of the lesson, the typical invitation to raise your hand and commit your life to loving and following Christ felt different. I felt like the Sunday school teacher was talking directly to me.

I looked around the circle of kids I sat with to see if they were feeling the same and shared my thoughts. But their faces were not flushed like mine, and they were not squirming in their seats as I was. I was disappointed to see them doing what I typically did at this time during the class: twiddling their hands, twirling their hair, and fiddling with their clothes. Finding no one who seemed to feel as I did, my heart began to beat faster and faster and pounded harder and harder in my chest. My ears felt hot and echoed like they were full of water. I had an overwhelming thought that I should raise my hand, but I did not know what to do next.

Suddenly, I recalled one of the many conversations I'd had with my cherished grandmother. I could hear her soothing voice as though she were sitting beside me, telling me about the Holy Spirit:

"God caused your heart, your brain, your lungs, and your Spirit to form when you were growing inside your mom's stomach. Your Spirit is the part of you attached directly to God. It is connected by an invisible but very strong, unbreakable cord that connects you to Him forever. He also placed His spirit, the Holy Spirit, inside of you too.

"The Holy Spirit is a part of God and knows all about you, even the parts you don't share. Think of the Holy Spirit as the part of God that is your best friend, the one that comforts and guides you in God's truth.

"The Holy Spirit understands God's language because it is a part of God. God's language and the way He communicates is much more advanced than ours. Not only does God speak every language in the world, He also created the languages for all the animals on Earth. So it is no surprise that God also speaks to us through our Spirit and in our thoughts. The Holy Spirit translates the messages from God to us. When the Heavenly Father speaks directly to you and calls on you, your Spirit will receive the message and help you to understand the instructions.

"The Holy Spirit knows and feels all things you feel. It communicates with you through the feelings and thoughts you have that tell you right from wrong and distinguish kindness and love from meanness. You know the feeling you get when you are doing something you shouldn't? You feel nervous about it and your heart may beat a little fast, and your hands may get a little sweaty, and then you get the feeling, like a nudge, that changes your mind. That is the Holy Spirit speaking to you and moving you toward what God wants for you.

"The Holy Spirit always tells you what God wants you to know. You will know it is the Holy Spirit speaking to you because it always leads you closer to God and toward God's goodness. The Holy Spirit will never tell you to do something wrong or hurt anyone's feelings. The Holy Spirit gives messages from God to your Spirit through your thoughts and gives your messages back to God. When we pray out loud or in our thoughts God hears us because of the Holy Spirit.

"When God is telling you to do something you've never done before, it will be very important. He will give the message to the Holy Spirit and he will give you God's instructions. He will stir your feelings up inside you, causing you to feel different or a little strange on the inside to get your attention. Your heart may beat rapidly, you may feel anxious or nervous, or you may feel hot, and you may feel like you have butterflies in your stomach. These feelings are like an alarm that something is going on.

"You will have an urgent thought that there is something you must do. I don't know what that will be. But in time you will know, because the Holy Spirit will make it very clear and tell you exactly what you should do.

"As God's interpreter, the Holy Spirit will send God's messages to you and from you to God for the rest of your life. So when you receive a message from God stirring inside, listen for His instructions. Do not be afraid. Do exactly what God is telling you to do."

Remembering what my grandmother told me, I knew I had to listen and respond to my overwhelming thoughts and emotions because the Holy Spirit was speaking to me. I had to make sure God knew that I loved Him and I heard Him.

Shyly, I raised my hand, and the Sunday school teacher called on me. I said I wanted to get baptized and show the Lord I love Him. Soon after I professed my intentions, my heartbeat slowed, my ears stopped ringing, the blood that rushed to my face faded, and I was flooded with happiness. The teacher smiled and said that was wonderful, but I had to talk to my parents first. I was so excited. I couldn't wait to tell my grandmother what happened.

I ran home as fast as my skinny eight-year-old legs could carry me to tell my parents and grandmother about the amazing event at church. They were proud that I made the choice to get baptized. My grandmother said she was not surprised; she knew I was special. I told them I was a little afraid because I was feeling so strange—hot, nervous, and confused. But I'd raised my hand anyway because it was like I was being called on, like a nudge to say "Yes" to the question: "Do you want to give your life to Christ? Do you accept that He is the Son of God and your Lord and Savior?"

My grandmother continued to prepare me for my life with Christ. She said there would be times when my Spirit would be filled with so much love that it would bubble inside me until it overflowed on the outside as singing, dancing, tears, or shouting, "I love you God." I shouldn't be shy about those big feelings of love because that is how we glorify God. I asked what that meant. She said, "Darling, that is just another word that means showing thankfulness and love toward the Lord our God." She emphasized that after my baptism it would be important to spend time talking and listening to God through His word in the Bible so that my Spirit and His Spirit would remain close. Just as best friends and family talk to each other every day, I should talk and listen to God daily.

On the day of my baptism, I was very excited, because I was telling God—and what seemed like thousands of church members—that I believe in God, that I believe He loves me, and I would always follow His instructions for what I should do.

At such a young age I didn't realize this vow of love that I sealed by saying, "Yes I believe and accept Jesus Christ as my Lord and Savior," would reinforce the invisible, unbreakable cord that connects God to me. I could not know then that my "Yes" would be the tether that would save my life from chronic pain and depression.

～

Spending time with my two siblings enriched my life, especially during rocky periods in my childhood. When my parents divorced, we spent a few weekends a month with my Dad. Living in Texas, we were never bothered by the summer heat. Throughout the neighborhood, we played tag and hide-and-seek, rode bikes, and kept cool running through the sprinklers and playing on the Slip 'N Slide. One afternoon, I rode my favorite pink bike with its multicolored plastic strings dangling from the handlebars in the alley driveway. The house directly across from our driveway was also on a downward sloping incline, creating a perfect V-shaped ramp in the alley.

The exhilaration of gaining speed going down one incline and up the other was the highlight of my yo-yo-like bike ride. I went up and down and back and forth. But the amusement abruptly ended when the front wheel of my bike collided with the front end of a speeding car. The next thing I recall was my sister crying and my brother yelling, "Are you okay?" My Dad was bent over me. As he picked me up, I felt the sting from hot concrete pebbles on the back of my arms, legs, and feet. Wrapping me in a blanket, he placed me in the backseat of the car and rushed me to the hospital.

My brother told me I was in the air as high as the roof and that my bike and sandals went up in the air too. According to the doctor, surviving this accident without a concussion, broken bones, or internal injuries was a miracle. This would be the second time I'd been told I was the recipient of a miracle.

When I was growing up, the adults in my family would tell me my life was miraculous because I was born prematurely at a time when the mortality rate for premature infants was high. I had a 50/50 chance of surviving, and if I survived, I had a 25% chance of having a permanent handicap. At three pounds, two ounces, I spent the first three months of my life in an incubator. At six years old, the story of my birth did not resonate much.

However, at age nine, I identified with the miraculous car accident. The ER doctor compared the impact of my body on the concrete to a drinking glass falling off a counter onto the floor. I'd seen shattered pieces of glass, and I was thankful my bones were not broken like it.

This accident would be the beginning of my walk alone with Christ, the beginning of difficult times that only I would experience, with my loved ones as observers. My older siblings, who always took care of me, couldn't protect me as they typically did from getting hit by the speeding car. Nor were there any adults who could prevent me from crashing onto the ground. This experience and the ones that followed began to awaken my awareness of the goodness of the God that my grandmother spoke about.

When divorce ripped the pages from my storybook childhood and poverty, sexual assault, and the impact of drug addiction on our family trailed a few years behind, the white picket fence of my youth was bulldozed. During my teenage years I was introduced to the reality that God does not always prevent deplorable things from happening, but with Him, getting through them is possible.

I knew for sure that it was only God who had protected me from the tragedies I encountered throughout life. However, it was not until the battle for my mental, physical, and spiritual well-being ensued that I learned what survival, resolute faith, and the mercy of God were all about.

CHAPTER THREE

The Plan

a strategy to achieve a goal

Three days after the definitive diagnosis, I saw the pain management doctor (also called a pain management specialist) recommended by the neurosurgeon. This type of medical doctor has had additional training to help patients manage severe pain. But not all pain management specialists have the same education and training.

There are two types of pain management doctors: interventional pain management and medical pain management. Many interventional pain management doctors spend several years learning advanced procedures and anesthesiology methods. They provide interventional procedures such as spine injections, epidurals, and nerve block implants in the spine that block pain at the nerve's site.

Medical pain management doctors generally prescribe pain medications and provide only minimally invasive steroidal injections in various areas of the body, excluding the spine. Their diverse medical backgrounds include, but are not limited to, internal medicine, neurology, orthopedics, and physical medicine and rehabilitation (PM&R), also known as physiatry.

My doctor was an interventional pain management doctor, a certified pain medicine anesthesiologist. This means he had extensive skills and specialized training to treat complex back, nerve, and cancer pain.

His plan involved giving me one, but no more than three, epidural spinal injections and a non-opioid pain medication. He would inject a steroid medication and a local anesthetic like lidocaine into my lumbar spine at the location of the bulging disc. This is a common approach on the conservative, no-surgery intervention plan to treat severe acute back pain. I was reassured by this treatment plan. My team, a neurosurgeon and pain management anesthesiologist, were also optimistic. We all agreed that I could expect the best possible outcome because I was "youngish," in perfect health, and in good physical shape. I felt both relieved and blessed to have experts on board who could steer me out of this situation.

The interlaminar injection was the first type of injection I'd receive. The doctor uses a fluoroscopy, a type of X-ray that enables him or her to see the location of the epidural needle when it is injected into the spine. This technique is called guided imaging, the precaution that ensures the needle is positioned correctly. The space where the needle is inserted is about 9 mm to 12 mm wide, the size of a kernel of corn. Thus, inserting the epidural needle too deep or just 1 mm to the right or left could result in adverse complications. He had to avoid puncturing the bulging disc and touching the irritated nerve causing my pain. Even with this microscopic margin of error and knowing the risks, my pain was too intense to pass on the possibility of relief. Having steroids injected in the exact location of the source of my pain bolstered my confidence that relief and a full recovery were just around the corner.

The day of the procedure, I accepted assistance to sit on the exam table and lie on my stomach. The procedure took fifteen to twenty minutes and began with numbing the injection site. I didn't feel the pinch of the needle, but I did feel a cramping pressure in my lower back as the needle was inserted deeply into my spine. The additional discomfort was a minor trade-off to achieve relief. I welcomed the injection—the first step to recovery, and a needed break from the havoc the bulging disc was wreaking on my body and my life.

During each follow-up appointment, the pain management doctor (Dr. P) repeatedly stated: "It's common to need more than one injection to achieve optimal relief." I appreciated him preparing me for the possibility of a minimal outcome from the initial injection.

Two weeks later, the frequency of the spasms and pain had marginally lessened, but not enough to resume normal living. I had been taking the prescribed anti-seizure medication, Lyrica, commonly used to treat nerve pain. Although, I took it several times a day, it did not lessen the pain.

Three weeks later came injection number two and a different prescription. He prescribed Gabapentin, another anti-seizure medication used for nerve pain and instructed me to stop taking the Lyrica. He dutifully reminded me to take the medication on schedule, increase the dosage as he prescribed, and to "stay ahead of the pain"—as if that was attainable with constant pain.

The second injection was a bilateral transforaminal injection. He warned it could cause more "discomfort" in the following days after the procedure because instead of one injection, I would have two. To administer the steroid, he'd insert a needle on either side of my vertebrae for the medication to have a greater impact on the pain. This was a gamble I was willing to take because I couldn't yet resume living my normal life. Betting on the sound medical advice and my general good health, I rolled the dice and hoped this injection would work.

The results, "more discomfort," was the myth my trusted advisor, Dr. P., sold me. I'd thought I was in terrible shape before. Sadly, it did not compare to what I experienced from the bilateral injections. For the next four days, I was in tears throughout the day and most of the nights due to spams and intensified sharp, electrocuting pains from my lower back to my feet. Two weeks after the injection, I still could only lie in bed or on the couch. Sitting in a chair for a meal was impossible. After the first injection, I could occasionally sit on a dining table chair for about twenty minutes a couple of times a week.

I had not anticipated this surprise setback, especially since I followed the medical advice to the letter. Dr. P. and the neurosurgeon agreed: My response was less than optimal, but it had always been a possibility for the pain to worsen. Dr. P. explained that the injection must have increased the inflammation; I needed to give my nerves more time to calm down.

The initial plan was not looking good; I was still so far from the goal. I'd arrived at the ten-week mile marker on my road to recovery, only two weeks beyond the estimated eight-week timeframe for me to return to work. Yet I was still unable to do the basic activities of daily living. I could not stand for more than ten minutes at a time or sit upright on the couch with my feet on the floor for longer than fifteen minutes. The least painful position was lying on my side or on my back with pillows to support the weight of my legs. The grip of pain was crushing my usual readily available optimism, and my confidence was beginning to vanish.

I was now the recipient of the empathy I had so freely given my patients. I was losing my sense of control over my condition. No longer a collaborator with my interdisciplinary team of physicians, nurses, and therapists, I was now a "true patient"—lying on the exam table waiting for my doctors to cure me, to save me. They were sympathetic to my sudden disabled condition. They often echoed one another, as if they were speaking with the same voice at the same time, saying the words

I've said so often to my patients: "I know this can be difficult, having to slow down, but recovery takes time."

Holding onto positivity by a thread as additional options for various procedures were being considered, I looked to them to infuse my waning confidence with hope. Disappointingly, there were few alternatives. Surgery with the possibility of more surgery as I got older, stronger pain medications, and the "Hail Mary": injection number three. My doctors thought it was still relatively early on my injury timeline. But was it? I wasn't sure which timeframe they meant, because we'd discussed six to eight weeks. I was supposed to see notable improvement along the way, yet none of that had happened. They backed away from the assurances they'd initially given me, as if I wouldn't notice. I'd been knocking on the door for recovery for three months. Yet my doctors answered only with euphemisms when they said: "You will get better soon. It is just taking longer for you to turn the corner. Bulging discs can be unpredictable. Just be patient."

What I heard was: "Be *a* patient." So I did what every patient in their right mind does—got a second opinion by consulting Dr. Google. Like my physicians, Dr. Google estimated the same six to eight weeks. I disregarded the articles that mentioned preexisting medical conditions—being overweight or having degenerative joint disease or an autoimmune condition—that would delay recovery, because those did not apply to me.

The unusual lack of improvement I was experiencing coupled with gnawing pain in my back, butt, legs, and feet fueled my frustration and worry. Opting for the less invasive spinal injections instead of surgery was my attempt to be reasonable, but reason was evaporating like dew under a blistering sun. My recovery was becoming more complicated, and hope was fleeing.

I was on the pain management train, taking an assortment of medications at various dosages and times, hoping they would lessen my symptoms. My days were consumed with managing my pain. Or, more accurately, my days were filled with my pain managing me. I couldn't get out of bed until took I took pain medication, and I couldn't do that until I ate, and I had to eat lying on my back because it hurt too much to sit up. Once the frequency of the spasms eased up, I was able to pursue other, nonpharmaceutical remedies to get through the day.

I spent hours in a hot bath of Epsom salt to alleviate the constant agony. It momentarily helped, and I could finally emerge to start my day of lying on the couch or bed. This cycle repeated daily, then weekly, then monthly. The earnest medical advice became a deflated lifeboat, and I was slowly drowning with no general timeframe of recovery to hold on to.

Once a month I had telehealth calls with the neurosurgeon. I was thankful I did not have to endure the painful car ride to his office, because every bump in the road caused a ferocious shock to suddenly course through my body. But the appointments with Dr. P. were every two weeks—in person. Both of their messages remained the same: "It may get better as time goes on. Some people respond well to this treatment, and some don't. You will just have to wait and see."

I also heard what they did not say, and it was steering me to a very dark place: "Get used to being on this end of the chronic back pain line because there's not much more we can do for you other than offer you more prescriptions or surgery. Your condition is likely permanent."

I felt like a dangling piece of bait on the end of a fishing line, waiting for this new way of life to devour me. With the original, definitive plan becoming a one of trial-and-error, the person I once knew as me was becoming less recognizable.

So terrified was I by the results of the second injection that I could not bring myself to go through with the third one Dr. P. was recommending. I was, however, willing to swallow his suggestion to take a higher dosage of Gabapentin three times a day, along with 1000 mg of Tylenol and 800 mg of Motrin three times a day.

My quality of life was slipping away. I didn't know how to stop the gravitational pull of my injury. The person who planned for everything that mattered in life, including college, career, marriage, and having children, could not plan for what was coming next. I was caught off-guard, blinded by the sudden attack of severe back pain on my life.

CHAPTER FOUR

Failed Plan

not achieving or falling short of the goal

It is astounding how severe pain can destroy everything in its path, like a blazing fire consuming a field of brush. In addition to my career and daily life, the pain ravaging my body was also consuming my family, my way of life, my peace, my hope, and my joy. I could not make plans until I consulted the pain, and neither could my family.

It was going to be yet another evening that moved along in slow motion for me and at a normal speed for them. Preparing dinners for my family, as well as their lunches, accompanied by fruity kale smoothies, had abruptly ended. The cheerful sounds of smooth jazz that set the rhythm for our busy evenings in the hub of our house, the kitchen, were replaced by dull chatting from the TV.

I hated the thought of my son finding me in my usual place, the bedroom, when he got home from high school. So lying on the couch before he arrived was my daily goal and a way to be present in our family's weekday routine.

One day around five o'clock I heard him enter the hallway. Pausing on his way to the kitchen, he chipperly asked, "Mom, do you think your back will be well enough for you to attend my wrestling tournament this week?"

I welcomed his preoccupation with dropping his lunch bag and water bottle in the sink and grabbing a snack. It gave me time to prepare a response that would neither shatter his optimism nor reveal my despair. We both had the same expectation for my recovery: that it would occur sooner rather than later.

Approaching the couch where where I lay, his mouth full of granola and yogurt, he poignantly added, "You missed the last two."

I hoped he wasn't tallying my absences from his matches, but I knew deep down he was keenly aware that things weren't improving. I wasn't back at work, nor was I making his favorite foods from scratch each evening. My heart was heavy.

Concealing the weight of the failed recovery plan, I lightheartedly responded, "I'm sorry, Son. You know those tournaments last four to seven hours and I still can't sit that long. I also need to lie down often to take the pressure off my back, and my doctor doesn't want me to climb gym bleachers yet."

With his usual carefree stride, he walked over to me. As he looked down at me from the foot of the couch, I saw the determination etched in the curves of his face. With the confidence of a winning attorney making his closing statement, he litigated his case for my attendance. "You can just sit on one of the folding chairs we usually sit in at the track meets during the summer and just stay on the gym floor," he said. "Then you won't have to climb the bleachers. When you need to, you can stand from time to time. You can also go out to the truck and recline in the seats so you can stretch out."

I didn't want him to know how impossible it would be for me to suppress my groans of pain when the car drove over the smallest bump in the road—or that I couldn't physically withstand the 90-minute round-trip ride without tears revealing what I was determined to conceal: The pain was defeating me.

I wasn't going to disappoint him by explaining the likelihood that I'd miss his entire freshman season. I needed to spare him my broken heart and camouflage my resentment about my injury to preserve his excitement for the season. So I feigned what I hoped would resemble a smile and begrudgingly responded, "Those chairs just don't give me enough support right now, so it won't be comfortable."

As he sat on the hearth of the fireplace near the end of the couch I was lying on, a self-assured chuckle punctuated his satisfaction at finding another solution to counter my excuse for skipping his match.

"Mom," he said, "we can obviously buy a different kind of chair for you."

When I briefly paused to show the consideration his thoughtful ideas warranted, my thoughts drifted. I wished his logic could solve my physical dilemma and that a different chair could suppress the pain.

Swallowing my bitterness, I cringed internally and sweetly said, "Maybe I can make the next match in a couple of weeks."

Sighing, he conceded. "Okay, Dad can record it for you. Or if the signal is good enough, he can FaceTime you so you can watch me live."

I was the one smiling now, because I could genuinely agree with him. I was glad he'd come up with an idea to resolve our impasse. During this round of our debate, my genuine delight returned to my voice as I said, "Sweetie, that's a great idea!"

Everything I considered doing had to be approved by my pain, the new authority in my life. Pain dictated the places I could go, what I did, and when I did it. I had to say farewell to date night, restaurant dining, museum trips, attending concerts, and after-dinner strolls. Pain, the thief that stole the pleasure in my life, was calling the shots, and I had to comply.

~

Looking out the window, I could see what used to be my vegetable garden. The vacant mound of dirt personified my physical condition and desolate state of mind. The lack of budding plants confirmed that there would be no organic grown mustard and collard greens on the menu for the upcoming holiday dinners.

My son's fifteenth birthday and Thanksgiving were approaching fast. Having only a few family members over for Thanksgiving dinner had not been unusual since the COVID pandemic normalized small family gatherings. But it would be unusual for me to not bake a delicious gluten- and dairy-free cake like the ones my son grew up with before we discovered he had food allergies.

It was obvious I was in no condition to prepare the annual elaborate holiday meal. Two weeks before my son's birthday, he sat on the couch beside me and asked how I was feeling. The conversation eventually got to the main topic he wanted to discuss: his birthday. He asked, "Do you think you'll to be able to make a cake for my birthday?"

He stared at me. The amber light in the living room illuminated the childlike hopefulness in his eyes, but his apprehension was apparent while he waited for my reply. His uncertainty called to me as his cries had when he was an infant. My heart raced and my personal fears and pain momentarily disappeared as my need to console and comfort him became my priority.

Although his 5'8" athletic build showed no indication of his need to be emotionally embraced, I had to ease his concern.

My motherly instincts took over. I needed to ensure my injury wouldn't disrupt his life any further. I wasn't going to allow this pain to bully or steal any more from my family. With my adrenaline spiking, I did not hesitate to answer him. Even if I had to alternate sitting or lying down and standing for three minutes at time or take several days to finish, I was going to the keep our seven-year tradition and bake his birthday cake. I reached for his hand, returned his intent gaze, and responded, "Of course, Sweetheart. Which of your favorite flavors do you want this year?"

The next tradition I was committed to uphold was turning our house into a winter wonderland with Christmas cheer in every corner and on every shelf. I had to somehow decorate the entire house from my bed and couch. I couldn't ask my son to pitch in beyond his usual duties of getting the decorations out of the attic. That would bring more attention to my lack of progress, and I wanted to spare us both from another debate-like discussion.

It wasn't unusual for some of my nieces to visit for several hours. So I enlisted one of them to help. This fun-filled day of Christmas decorating included tasty store-bought appetizers, mocktails for me, and festive cocktails for her.

I was thankful for her agility. She climbed the ladder and stood on top of the counters to place the ornate reindeers, decorative sleds, jolly snowmen, glittered red and gold poinsettias, and tinseled angels above the kitchen cabinets and in various nooks. She patiently placed all the ornaments on the 10-foot-tall warm-lit Christmas tree. The sounds of "A Charlie Brown Christmas" by the Vince Guaraldi Trio and other traditional songs were the soundtrack for the merry day. In that moment, my favorite holiday briefly lifted my spirits, momentarily freeing me from the burden of my troubles.

Waking up to the New Year, I began to ponder when this injury began to rewrite the story of my life. It was right after the leaves abandoned the trees cracks began to form in my hope. Staring at the frost on the grass, I began to accept the condolences of my physicians and continued to do what my body demanded: chase the notion of becoming pain free. The Gabapentin I took to pacify the pain caused me to sleep more hours than I was awake. Although this wasn't the picture of recovery, what else could I possibly do?

A thousand questions flooded my mind with no apparent answers. What happens when the body is no longer under your control? When physical pain induces psychological pain? How could I escape this emotional bondage?

The shock of physical pain was colluding against the intangible hope and faith imbued in my Spirit. The ceaseless incantation from my pain in my body and mind went something like this: "Putting an end to the pain is a good thing. It's not good to suffer. You should be as close to pain free as possible. You can't recover if your body is stressed by constant pain. Don't worry, the side effects from the prescription are only a small sacrifice in an exchange for relief and recovery."

The half-truths my body was peddling had me convinced I was doing the right thing by taking the prescriptions on schedule at the prescribed doses. This prevented the pain from escalating to its highest peak. Additionally, sleeping is resting, which is best for recovery.

At my ninth follow-up doctor's appointment, the severity of my pain was dutifully affirmed, and the futile plan of treatment continued. Although I was talking to Dr. P., the neurosurgeon also echoed his message when I had my appointments with him. They both said:

"Paula, as a therapist you know nerve pain is the worst kind of pain. Don't overdo it when your pain level is less. You know you'll make your symptoms worse. Right now, managing the symptoms is the best thing we can do for you, and it's the best thing you can do for yourself. Take it easy, don't push yourself, and take the meds as scheduled."

Their endorsement for this ineffective treatment plan swayed me to accept as truth the blood-curdling scream from my body and mind: "GIVE ME RELIEF. NO MATTER THE COST!". And I obeyed.

Despite my spiritual, professional, and collegiate wherewithal, the illusive plan ushered me into a state of denial, anger, and depression. I was in denial about the permanence of my condition. This prolonged my inability to pivot to a sustainable recovery plan that would guarantee a positive emotional perspective. I was unraveling emotionally and I did not have the capacity to step outside my patient status to be the therapist I had been for my patients.

As recovery evaded me, the bargaining I was doing worsened my state of mind. I bargained with myself that altering the number of pills I took and doing small things around the house was proof that I was improving. When that failed, I became even angrier: Nothing I did reduced the pain, healed my back, or met my expectations of a 90% chance of full recovery. My doctors could not offer me more reassurance in my stalled recuperation. I was angry because I did not want to consider what my life would look like if I didn't fully recover. I was emotionally defeated because I could not see a way out from under the pressure of this bulging disc. My life consisted of pills, the bed, the couch, and the tub. I existed nowhere else.

Once my anger lessened and the shock of "this is really happening to me" wore off, I accepted that the plan was not working. Depression and defeat took turns ripping holes in my psyche, and I was overwhelmed by having to consider ending a twenty-year career and permanently alter how I lived my life. As grief engulfed me, I was too ashamed to share my truth and guilty that the relentless assault of pain and depression overshadowed my friends' and family's continual encouragement.

I did my best to smile and act optimistic for the sake of my loved ones. How could I admit that I was lonely and defeated when they were doing their best to help me? It would have been cruel and selfish to let on that their heartfelt expressions of compassion—kind words, text messages and phone calls—only brushed the surface of my internal misery.

No amount of love and empathy from them could ease my physical and mental distress. It broke my heart to see how hard they tried. They were in my corner supporting me, but I was the only person in the ring who could fight this battle for my life. Although I was loosing daily, I was too ashamed to share my truth.

The adage of "fake it until you make it" became my mantra. I wanted and needed to feel better for them. I did not want to project how miserable I felt or burden them with my grief.

I longed for the cheerfulness I projected to quell the darkness inside me. Some days I was afloat on their love and assurances. But more often the darkness won out. I was slipping below the surface of life and I did not want to complain too much or spew the negativity that flooded my innermost thoughts. It would make them feel uncomfortable and powerless to hear me say, "I feel dismal, I'm riddled with anxiety, and by the way: I AM HURITNG ALL THE TIME and IT NEVER ENDS!"

I could not do much, but I could try to lessen their concern with a display of positivity, and I took off my mask of optimism only when alone behind the closed doors of the bathroom. I surrendered to my pain in the warm salt bath. In there I wept and emptied my soul of my mental and physical anguish. It was there that I soaked in tears of despair. But when I emerged, I performed the "I'm feeling better show," hoping it would someday be true. This included standing up while making a sandwich or sitting on the couch folding clothes. I tried to feel better, and for a moment I did, and I was able to brush off the physical setbacks that remanded me to bed even longer on the following days.

Eventually, though, I became the prisoner of the coercive arm of chronic back pain. The strength I once had to put on optimism and hide my depression for the sake of my loved ones was annihilated in the fight for my soul. I became an empty vessel of hope.

CHAPTER FIVE

The Edge

the brink; the threshold
of something; the boundary

During my tenth visit, my doctor asked for the third or fourth time if I'd try a low dose of Tramadol, a synthetic opioid. I remained resistant to his offer. Perhaps he thought he was being kind, trying to help alleviate my pain. But through the filter of my life experiences, I heard him say, "Do you want to try a low dose of opioid addiction for a little while to see if your quality of life improves?" Frustrated that he had not heard or remembered my stance on opioids, my tight-lipped response was a firm "No." Inside, I was shouting, "Are You Crazy? Absolutely Not!"

According to the Drug Enforcement Administration's (DEA) classifications of drugs used for medical purposes that have the potential for abuse, Tramodol (Schedule IV) is considered less habit-forming than Tylenol with Codeine #3 (Schedule III) and significantly less than Hydrocodone (Schedule II).

The Controlled Substance Schedule, commonly referred to as The Schedule, is a classification used by the DEA, pharmacists, and physicians to categorize drugs, substances, and chemicals used to make legal and illegal substances or drugs with potential psychological and/or physical dependence. They're called "controlled substances" because the government closely regulates or "controls" how the highly addictive or abusive substance in the medication is stored, dispensed, and manufactured.

The Schedule is divided into five categories: Schedule I, II, III, IV, and V, arranged in descending order based on the prevalence for abuse/dependency. I and II have the greatest potential abuse/addiction and V has the least. Subcategories in Schedule II and III substances include non-opioid prescriptions, which are referred to as 2N and 3N.

There is only one difference between Schedule I and Schedule II drugs. Schedule I are illicit substances like heroin and Ecstasy. Schedule II substances are prescribed by a doctor. Schedule II drugs include Vicodin, Methadone, Dilaudid, Oxycodone, Hydrocodone, Norco, Fentanyl, Adderall (2N), and Ritalin (2N).

The controlled substances on Schedule III "have a moderate or low potential for physical dependence or a high psychological dependence"[14]. These medications include Suboxone (buprenorphine/naloxone), Tylenol 3, and other products containing less than 90 milligrams of codeine per dose, such as ketamine (3N) and anabolic steroids (3N).

Schedule IV controlled substances such as alprazolam (Xanax®), carisoprodol (Soma®), clonazepam (Klonopin®), clorazepate (Tranxene®), diazepam (Valium®), and lorazepam (Ativan®), represent a lower potential for abuse and a lower risk of physical dependence compared to Schedule III substances, but they all carry a risk for psychological dependence.

Schedule V medications/substances have the least potential for abuse and physical and/or psychological dependence. They contain limited quantities of narcotics (less than 200 milligrams of codeine), or no narcotics. Cough medications like Robitussin AC contain 10 mg of codeine. Additional medications in this category are antidiarrheal medications like Lomotil and Lyrica, a non-opioid medication with multiple uses, including lessening anxiety, seizures, and pain. A similar medication to Lyrica, Gabapentin (brand name Neurontin), is not a controlled substance according to the DEA. However, Kentucky, Michigan, West Virginia, Alabama, and Tennessee regulate Gabapentin as a Schedule IV controlled substance due to an increase in illicit use[15,16].

~

Seeing the toll of addiction in lives of my patients and other members of my family was the primary reason I was determined to reject prescription narcotics. Having a front-row seat to the demise of one of the most loved and influential human beings in my life as a result of a relationship with addictive "party" substances made me emphatically refuse the mere suggestion of medications similar to Oxycodone.

I watched the person who set my standards for how capable, intelligent, and loving a man should be, slowly disintegrate from a towering 6'3" muscular alpha male with chubby cheeks and a round protruding midsection showing the signs of his love for food permanently changed my relationship with addiction forever.

His warm smile was accented by his full beard and the sweet peppery scent of Old Spice cologne. The strength and power of his arms was accentuated by his above average 6'5" wingspan; the length and span of his hands rivaled a seven-foot-tall NBA basketball player's. His agility and speed playing a competitive game of basketball, flag football, or ping-pong at the community rec center and park were as surprising as a 6'11" linebacker doing a grand jete ballet maneuver over an opponent ready to tackle him.

The witty jack-of-all-trades endearingly called "Teddy" (short for Teddy Bear), was always orchestrating a prank to make you laugh—because "playing," as he would say in his smooth baritone voice, "is not just for kids." You could hear his love for life in his robust laugh and endless hilarious jokes that were borderline age-appropriate for us siblings and the neighborhood kids who adored him.

He walked with swagger, and his slight gap-toothed smile softened the fierceness of his jawline and intense deep-set eyes. People were drawn to his free-spirited personality and captivating presence. I always felt special because everyone's favorite son, brother, uncle, and friend was my Dad.

Seeing him slowly—and then quickly—shrink to an unrecognizable shell of the human being he once was, was seared into my 17-year-old mind. His bear-like stature diminished and his stout tree-trunk legs were reduced to saplings. Remembering the strength of the arms that tossed me effortlessly in the air as a child and cradled me when I was afraid disappeared. The light in his eyes and his formidable character could be seen only in my memory and in photographs from years past.

~

Considering the influence of the biological, environmental, genetic, and psychosocial factors, I recognized my risk for developing an OUD (opioid use disorder) or SUD (substance use disorder)[17]. However, environmental and psychosocial factors were not an issue for me. As an adult, I'd lived in a stable, healthy, drug-free home and community, had a rewarding career, a strong support system, a healthy outlet for stress, and a faith-based belief system.

It was the genetic and biological factors that placed me on the tight-rope of addiction. I had never undergone metabolic or genetic testing to determine if my baseline metabolic system that regulates mood was vulnerable to becoming dysregulated when taking controlled substances or mood-altering prescriptions[18].

My family history of depression, another leading factor that increases vulnerability to addictive substances, made me acutely aware of my risk. Having a first-degree relative, a parent, with an OUD meant I faced a 50% likelihood of developing an OUD or SUD. That statistic gave me grave pause[19]. For me, avoiding potentially addictive substances was more than a health-conscious choice. I had to strictly avoid potentially addictive medications, because the risks were too great.

The alternative prescriptions for opioids my doctor suggested were a class of medications called gabapentinoids. These are commonly pre-scribed to treat nerve pain, epilepsy, and fibromyalgia. They have a low threshold for inducing physical or psychological dependence if used as prescribed.

I agreed to take Lyrica (the Schedule V medication), and Gabapentin. When discussing the side effects with my doctor, I was not concerned by the major one he emphasized—drowsiness. I felt comfortable with the medication's non-habit-forming potential. I was also very familiar with these medications because over half of the chronic pain patients I encountered took them, along with other analgesics.

Lyrica and Gabapentin are pharmaceutical "downers" that can cause a euphoric, sedative feeling, induce sleep, and decrease anxiety—just like the non-pharmaceutical downer, alcohol. They're called "downers" because they decrease central nervous system activity. This part of the nervous system functions like a relay switch, instructing the body when to wake or sleep, when to physically or emotionally react to a situation, and when not to react.

These were the "safe" prescriptions I turned to aid my recovery. I would be only a tad drowsy, a manageable side effect. Only people who already suffered from OUD, SUD, or mental illness were at risk of developing an SUD from these medications. Additionally, I did not perceive Gabapentin as a risk factor that could impact my mental health[20].

I had a "strong mind "and I was aware of the signs of abnormal dependency and abuse. I was careful, I was cautious, and I followed my doctors' instructions. I would increase the medication every several days, just as prescribed.

My plan was to heal and eliminate the pain. I thought avoiding opioids and taking a medication that "only" quieted my overactive nervous system would insulate me from dysfunctional dependency. But I was fooling myself. I did develop an unhealthy psychological dependence on the pills. Pharmaceutically-induced sleep became my drug of choice. Gabapentin momentarily quieted the pain in my nervous system and my thoughts. It created a deadly hiding place for my distressed mind.

I was so focused on not falling into the trap of overt addiction, like taking the medication otherwise than prescribed, that I missed the million tiny cuts depression was etching into my soul, which made me vulnerable to psychological dependency. Gradually, I began to medicate my emotional pain, as so many others with an SUD or OUD do. Wanting to silence the noise from the psychological pain, I welcomed the side effect of being awake for just six to eight hours a day and convinced myself this was normal.

I followed the prescription schedule and waited for the chemical magic to dull my mental state. Although temporary, I longed for the veil of pseudo relief to fall and cover the grotesque edges of my emotional wounds. Taking the maximum dosage of the medication didn't lessen the physical pain; it changed into a sharp blade that made clean, defined puncture wounds instead of a jagged-edged blade that burned and shredded my insides with each breath.

I depended on sedation from the pills to lull me into an acceptable stupor that imitated rest. It was then that the voices of my pain, disappointment, depression, and fears berated me less. But after being awake for less than an hour, the serrated blade returned, and I waited for the next scheduled dose. I unconsciously placed my hope in a failed plan for my recovery.

During a routine visit to Dr. P., we discussed how my pain was doing—not how I was doing. I felt like a supporting character, with my pain being the star in this simulation for recovery.

I told him, "I'm taking 300 mg of the Gabapentin three times a day."

"How is that working for you?" he said.

"It only takes the edge off somewhat when I also take the maximum doses of Motrin, 800 mg three times a day, 1000 mg of Tylenol three times a day, and the muscle relaxer twice a day. But it doesn't lessen the pain enough for me to do normal things for myself and my family."

"The maximum dosage is 1200 mg three times a day. You're far from that amount. I want you to start taking an additional 100 mg in the morning to see if this decreases your symptoms. If not, we'll adjust at your next visit. The dosage of this medication is increased slowly to get to a therapeutic level effective for your pain."

Before I could respond, my husband's facial expression, suddenly changed. A deep wrinkled formed and protruded between his eyes, as if the frustration and concern he felt was searching for an outlet, but instead it was suppressed into the crevices of his forehead. His low, terse tone did not conceal his outrage at my doctor's suggestion.

"You are recommending she take more?" This sounded like an indictment as he slowly articulated each syllable. "She is sleeping a lot already from what she's taking. She barely wakes up to eat and is only awake for about five to six hours a day."

Dr. P.'s gaze flashed from my husband to me. He acknowledged my husband's concerns by folding his arms across his chest and nodding his head intently. Once he rediscovered his voice, he said in an unusually high pitch, "The medication does cause drowsiness."

My husband sarcastically said, "And you think being awake for six hours a day is normal?"

He didn't respond to my husband. Instead, using his most composed and authoritative voice, Dr. P said, "Paula, if you are bothered by how drowsy you feel, you can take less in the daytime and take up to 400 mg at night to help you sleep comfortably. Just be consistent with the schedule and the dose. Don't stop taking the Gabapentin suddenly, because you'll feel unwell."

This last statement should have sounded the alarm that the Gabapentin was not as harmless as I'd thought. His warning meant I'd have to be tapered off the prescription to avoid the physical withdrawal side effects associated with this medication. But it didn't register; my hopelessness was deafening, and I continued to take the counterfeit remedy in the prescription bottle.

~

"Sweetheart, you must wake up. It is almost two in the afternoon and you've had nothing to eat or drink. The crackers I left for you are still here," my husband said.

I slowly opened my eyelids, which felt like they weighed one hundred pounds, and saw the worry in his eyes. In a poor attempt to assuage his concern, I mumbled defensively, "I woke up and drank all the water you left on the nightstand."

It was easier to suffer in the confines of my bed. I was now taking enough of my medications at night to be able to sleep, albeit uncomfortably, until the afternoon. I no longer had the motivation to will myself to be a picture of perseverance and optimism. I was getting out of bed only for my husband and son's sake. If they were not present I can't say for sure I how long I would have remained in bed. On waking I disappeared in a warm salt bath for three to four hours until I could emerge for the Lights, Camera, Action, I'm Doing Better Show. But even this performance was becoming a thing of the past. More often, my son found me in bed when he returned from school instead of on the couch.

I couldn't fake positivity for even one more day. In my despair, I felt how easy it would be to slip away into a SUD by taking more and more pills. In my vulnerable state of mind, I was falling towards permanent desolation with futility as my only companion. I encountered the whisper that nudges one off the edge of hopelessness, and these thoughts terrified me.

My fears rampantly unfolded—as if I were watching myself in a remake of *A Christmas Carol*, the movie based on the novel by Charles Dickens. "The Ghost of Christmas Yet to Come" was visiting me, transporting me through scenes of my future as a shroud of depression and dysfunctional prescription dependency invaded my life.

First, the faceless figure escorted me on what appeared to be a regular day. I saw myself lying in bed awake. It was late in the afternoon because I heard the sport program that aired after 2:00 blaring from the living room. As I contemplated taking back control of my life, I decided to prepare a modified version of one of my family's favorite meals—fried chicken wings and macaroni and cheese from scratch. I could oven fry the chicken instead of standing at the stove and make a quick scratch mac and cheese. I could season the chicken and make the cheese sauce while sitting on a bar chair with good back support. I could ask my husband to place sheet pan with five pounds of chicken in the oven. I felt I could definitely do this.

But then, the sunlight in the room abruptly dimmed. Thunder and lightning rumbled outside, causing my bedroom windows to shake. As the voice of my pain filled the room my hands became sweaty, my throat was dry, and my heart raced.

As the ghostly figure looked on, my pain said, "Do you remember the last time you tried to overcome me and cooked dinner for your family to disregard me?"

"I do," I said. "You tormented me with bolts of spasms from my waist to the soles of my feet for two days in addition to the daily clenching pain around my waist. The spasms were twenty times worse than birthing contractions."

"I told you I'd make you regret your clever ideas. I tell you what you can do and when you can do it," my pain dictated. This menacing threat crushed my promising idea.

Instead of getting out of bed, I ate the crackers my husband left for me, took my pills, and went back to sleep.

Pain was the parasite that continued to gnaw at my life, causing it to become unrecognizable. I wasn't spending time outdoors enjoying nature, planting spring flowers, going bike riding, or sharing intimate moments with my husband. Who was this person who only slept, barely ate, took medication multiple times a day and did absolutely nothing productive? Where was the physically active person who occupied the helm of all things joyful and nurturing in my home, the person who facilitated healing in others? Pain had the upper hand, latching on to all aspects of my existence.

As my sorrow-tinged trance continued, my husband woke me from yet another early afternoon nap, saying, "It's beautiful outside, and the winds are just right for us to take the boat out on the lake." He added, "You haven't been to the lake the entire boating season and it will be ending soon."

I was burdened with guilt because boating was a favorite family hobby. Before I could courageously say that I'd get out on the lake this time—after I took my medication and soaked in the tub for just one hour—my overlord and fear answered for me, saying: "There's no way I can step off that floating pier onto the boat, or bear the constant sway of the waves. And I cannot walk on the incline down to the pier. That will aggravate my body way too much. I'll stay home and y'all can head to the lake."

As my husband turned to leave the bedroom, I shouted, "Wait! I want to go with you!" But my voice didn't make a sound. It was like nightmares I had where I screamed for help and no sound came out. I was left alone with my medication and despair to keep me company.

Then, the haunted guide gave me another glimpse of myself becoming a bystander in my life. The influence of the prescribed medications rendered me powerless and the pain cycle diminished the control I had over my life. I slept when I wanted to be awake and when I was awake, I was useless:

"Mom!" my son shouted, startling me out of an involuntary mid-day doze. What is wrong with you? You kept falling asleep while I was telling you what happened at school today, and you never answered me about the grilled cheese sandwich."

"I'm so sorry, Son. You can finish telling me about your day when you get out of the shower. I'll make your sandwich." But after he'd showered, I was lying on the couch asleep. I never made it to the kitchen.

I desperately wanted to hear everything he had to say and be a part of my family dynamic. But I had become a victim of the side effects from my emotional injuries. My judgment was sidelined by the stealthy influence of pain and depression. The constant pressure and stress from pain would thrust my mind and body into a fight-or-flight mode, bypassing calculated reasoning, and only seeking the most efficient means to alleviate the pain. I was petrified by these distraught scenes.

The grisly figure showed me the date on my phone: It was winter, three years later, and my son's senior year in high school. More prescriptions had been added to my daily regimen: Hydrocodone (Schedule II) and Valium (Schedule IV), for anxiety. Old faithful Gabapentin and the muscle relaxer remained on my nightstand. I panicked seeing those prescription bottles, but I could not stop my look-alike from reaching for them and taking her daily dose.

The pain relief and the promise of recovery in the bottle is deception at its finest. I observed myself willingly take part in the ploy of healing and recovery. Watching the clock with each dose I took, I waited for the three hours to pass so I could re-up. My hope and my life were trapped in the bottle. The neon warning signs of opioid use disorder were now in my rearview; pain invaded every waking moment. Stopping it was my only goal. The caution I once so carefully deployed faded as desperation for a respite from the relentless onslaught of emotional and physical pain set in. I was taking more pills per day than what was written on the bottles.

Gently shaking me on my shoulder, my son said, "Hey Mom, are you awake? Do you think you're going to make it to my match tomorrow? There are only two left in my final season."

"Of course. I'm taking a different medication, and it is working really good. I'll definitely be there," I said.

"You haven't made it to any of my matches for the last three years. Are you sure you're going to come? It's senior night and everyone's parents will be there," he added.

I wasn't taking a different medication, just a higher dose, but I couldn't let him know that. I was determined to assure him that I'd be there. I added caffeine pills and energy drinks to my diet to keep me awake.

I easily understood how addiction had become a bartered compromise in exchange for a moment of silence from the relentless physical and emotional pain. I had an OUD (opioid use disorder). I was taking all my prescriptions at more frequent intervals than prescribed, using Valium and Gabapentin as I saw fit to make the effects of the Hydrocodone last longer, and I ignored the adverse effects my habit was having in my relationships.

With my eerie companion, I continued to visit Dr. P. to get my monthly supply. He asked the routine questions, and I gave the same stock answers and accepted the prescription for the controlled substances that were controlling me.

By taking one narcotic pill at a time, I stood at the doorway of addiction. But it wasn't until depression nudged me, that I walked through it—stumbled into the trap that awaited me at the end of my empty prescription bottles.

I was afraid for my son, my husband, and my entire family. They would lose a mother, wife, sister, aunt, daughter, and friend because I was tethered to pills and my bed. The thought of them living with a shadow of who I once was unbearable. The initial plan, one once paved with hope and healing, was now filled with addiction and loss. I had to get out of this doomed cycle. I wanted this tour through my doomed future to end. I had to get up from the bed that had become my living casket. I had to flee. But how?

My husband walked into our bedroom and sadly said, "It's been three years since you decorated the house for Christmas. Don't you want to have our home decorated with more than the reindeer on the table. You said you'd do it this year. That was two weeks ago, and Christmas is in two weeks. We would love to help. Or you could have one of our nieces over to help."

Before my doppelgänger responded, I saw myself wake up. I couldn't tell if it was night or day because the room was dark. I reached for my phone: the date was December 26. I'd slept through Christmas day and my family didn't bother to wake me.

I punched and kicked my silent phantom guide, demanding answers for what was happening to me; death was closing in. It remained silent, only pointing to the prescription bottles on my nightstand, my physician's number in my phone's recent call log, and my Bible.

The dreadful journey through my doomed future continued. In the next scene, I was confronted with the myths about people who suffer from opioid use disorder.

I said to a patient's nurse: "The patient I was scheduled to see for occupational therapy complained of back pain and asked for pain medication before getting out of bed."

The nurse replied in a dry tone, "Her chart shows a long history of opiate prescriptions and drug-seeking behavior. Apparently, some years ago she had a back injury and several back surgeries. She's here recovering from pneumonia and respiratory failure so there's nothing really wrong with her. She probably got hooked on painkillers and didn't stop taking them when she was supposed to. She has routine morphine, Gabapentin, a muscle relaxer, and Ativan to help with her pain and anxiety. She's taken them all. She'll need to wait an hour and a half before she can take her next scheduled dose. She's probably just trying to get out of doing therapy with you. I'll tell her she has to wait."

"Okay. Too bad she didn't avoid those opioids. Some people just don't take their medication as prescribed," I responded, not giving the patient a second thought.

But The Ghost of Christmas Yet to Come directed me back to the pain patient's room and pointed to photos on a shelf—pictures of her young grandchildren and vacation photos. As I tried to leave, the phantom forcibly turned me so I could see the photo of her family. It was blurred. But as I focused on the image, I recognized the woman in the photo—it was me.

I collapsed, falling endlessly, desperate to hit the ground so the impact would bring me back to reality. But the ghastly chaperon forced me to linger in torment and stare at the unrecognizable woman I had become.

Initially, everything the nurse told me seemed plausible, until I realized she was talking about me—the health conscious, God-fearing mother, daughter, wife, and therapist.

As a patient, I was seen as cunning and untrustworthy, and my complaints of pain were dismissed. The nurse and therapist blamed me for my dependency and labeled me as drug-seeking. Scrutiny and judgment prevailed over compassion. The stigma of Schedule II opioid pain medications was obvious in the nurse's remark, as was my indifference. I was disgusted by my lack of empathy and callous disregard.

A panorama of my treatment flashed before my eyes, starting with my first doctor's appointment and showing the many years that followed, highlighting the moments when depression began and doubt set in. I saw myself adopting the behaviors of someone with an OUD, misleading all around me. Despite how the pills and my depression caused me to withdraw from my life, I never asked for help. Instead, I hid behind Christian expressions like "God is Good," to conceal the truth and my humiliating defeat.

My phantom replayed all my unsuccessful attempts to lessen the medication doses. It exposed the contradiction I'd become: a Christian healthcare professional with an OUD, depression, and anxiety.

Standing with the Phantom outside my bedroom, looking in at myself lying in bed with six prescription bottles on my nightstand, I saw what my life could become if I continued to let pain and depression defeat me. I knew I was just another dose away from making these dark scenes reality. I begged the grim, hooded guide to end this nightmare of dread and shame.

Once my racing foreboding thoughts slowed, my phantom ruminations disappeared, and I could see myself more clearly. I was able to honestly ask myself, "How did I get into this anguished state of mind? How did I fall from the seat in Heaven that Christ gave me when I accepted him as Lord?"

CHAPTER SIX

Confrontation

defiantly facing your opponent

"Sweetheart," my husband affectionately said, "Are you doing okay? You've been in in this tub for a long time. I've had three conference calls in the last three hours. Have you been crying? You look like you have been crying. I'm going to cancel my next meeting and sit with you for a little while. Let me get a chair."

He asked and answered his own questions so rapidly that I didn't get a chance to respond until he returned with a folding chair.

As he sat, he exhaled a long breath. This was my cue to address his concerns. Smiling with my voice because I couldn't cajole it to reach my face, I said, "You don't have to do that. I'm fine. I am feeling a little low, but nothing for you to worry about."

He pleaded, "What can I do for you?" His words were gentle and caressed my face like the tear that trickled down my cheek. I wanted to reassure him and shield him from my despair, so I replied with a painted-on smile: "You're doing plenty by filling in for me around the house and with our son. I'll be fine." But my hopeful words neither comforted him nor concealed the melancholy that outlined my swollen, red-rimmed eyes.

He looked at me with a half-smile that tried to convey the optimism he wished he felt and could see in me. But his powerlessness was palpable, his broad shoulders and head lowered in a posture of defeat. The air was not just thick with humidity from the hot bath water; his dejected emotions along with mine filled the room. The mound of emotions clogging our throats made it difficult for us to utter a word. And our speechless sorrow mingled between our shared gaze. He leaned over to kiss my forehead. With his face close to mine, he stroked the back of my head and said, "I love you. Whatever you need, we are here for you."

Wishing I could disappear, I submerged my sullen body further into the warm water and managed to mimic in a chipper tone, "Honey," thank you. I'm fine. Soaking in the tub just takes some of the pressure off my back."

He leaned back in the chair with folded arms as our silent banter resumed. He continued to look at me compassionately yet intensely, waiting for me to confess what I was failing to hide. About thirty minutes later he exhaled again, ending the long uncomfortable pauses in our conversation. He reluctantly sighed "okay," and gave me another pensive smile. Then he stood and said, "I love you." He tenderly kissed me on the forehead again and walked out of the bathroom.

My attempt to project hopefulness as recompense for his concern during these frequent bathtub encounters kept missing the mark. I asked myself how many more times could I watch him retreat into his own helplessness. Seeing his worry was disheartening. The side effects of my injury was smothering the happiness of those I loved. I searched my soul to find a way to free myself and my family from the quicksand my condition trapped us in—but I did not find a solution.

~

It was the beginning of another forlorn week and the lavender scented water did not cover up the stench from my despondent state of mind. When I glanced outside the bathroom window, I couldn't help but notice that conditions outside mirrored those inside of me. The sun was shining, but it was 28 degrees and the leafless ice-covered branches resembled my frozen Spirit. Although the consoling hot bath was a haven from the frigid temperatures outside, it did nothing to provide an asylum for my battered soul. Despite my plastered-on radiant smiles to project contentment for family I remained frozen in my depression.

I stared at the steam rising from the water. The particles of dust were floating in the streams of light gleaming through the window. The shimmering sunlight filled the bathroom with an ambiance of calm—the opposite of the angst I was feeling. A brilliant ray poured through the top of the shutters, creating an immaculate beam of light where the ceiling and walls met, as if it were a spotlight shining directly from heaven to catch my attention.

Looking up, this beacon of light captivated my thoughts. My senses heightened. I could suddenly feel the sun's rays on the top of my bent knees. The tense muscles in my back began to relax as melodies of grace, mercy, and transformational power through surrender muffled the moaning coming from my injured soul.

My wounded faith was serenaded by God's unconditional love and faithfulness in ballads like *Isaiah Song* by Maverick City Music. Eventually, my Spirit peeped out from under my gloom to hear what my Lord was proposing in the anthems of hope and triumph that filled the room.

As one song ended and another began, my fragmented thoughts began to realign, and I was drawn to His mercy. Then I heard God call my name. Not the name my mother gave me, but the name He gave me: My Beloved Daughter, My Chosen and Blessed One. My surging tears answered His call. And He spoke these words to me:

This is not the place I had in mind for you to worship when I formed you in your mother's womb. Come out of this forsaken place. Walk in the Light.

Rejoin Me.

I never intended for you to leave my presence when this injury began.

But pain and fear have pulled your trust and your heart away from me.

Come back to the place I made for you. It is still beside Me.[*]

Trust Me.

Do not be afraid to stop taking the pills. The pain may howl, but I will sustain you.

My presence will restore you.

I am the God of comfort.

I am the God of compassion.[†]

Those pills are darkness, and they make it difficult for you to see Me clearly.

I am the light. And where light is, darkness cannot remain.

Reclaim your courage.

Come to Me.

Unplugging the blaring microphone from my pain, He silenced the pandemonium in my heart and my mind. My body shuddered and shook from the pounding, torrential tears that coursed through my soul and down my face. El Shaddai, the Almighty God, went on to have a more specific conversation with my Spirit. He said:

---

[*] John 14: 1-4 NIV My Father's house has many rooms . . . I am going there to prepare a place for you . . . I will come back and take you to be with me that you also may be where I am
[†] 2 Corinthians 1:3 NIV I am the God of compassion. I am the God of comfort.

I am uprooting your optimism because those are shallow roots in rocky soil. It produces only temporary peace and artificial hope. Optimism is not sustainable in the great suffering that occurs in the tribulations in life. Optimism is like a tent in the desert that can only provide shade from the blistering sun, but it will not withstand the ferocious winds of the sandstorms in life. The tent of optimism is a shred of thin fabric blowing in the wind.

Only the foundation and walls of true faith have the durability and structure to withstand all of life's storms. Faith is the shelter that covers you. It is the anchor that keeps you tethered to Me. It is your strong tower when you are in a battle. And my Beloved, you are in a battle for your soul, but I have fought for you. I am fighting this battle with you. And I have never lost a battle (Deuteronomy 20:4 NIV)‡. I have never left you, nor have I forsaken you. Do not be afraid. Do not remain discouraged (Deuteronomy 31:8).

Your optimism and positivity were the glue that held your faith together. Now that inadequate glue has come apart. I will rebuild your faith with the sustaining and substantial power that is in the truth of My Word. Remember what I have said about you and your circumstances. In your lifetime, in this world that you live in, you will have difficult times but be at peace because I have overcome the world (John 16:33 NIV). Do not throw away your confidence in Me because I will reward you and keep my promise to deliver you from the frightful battle you are in (Hebrews 10:35, Psalms 91:3–7 NIV)§.

---

‡ "For the LORD your God is the one who goes with you to fight for you against your enemies to give you victory."

§ Hebrews: So do not throw away your confidence; it will be richly rewarded.
Psalms: Surely, he will save you . . . He will cover you . . . you will find refuge; his faithfulness will be your shield.You will not fear the terror of the night . . . A thousand may fall at your side, ten thousand at your right hand, but it will not come near you . . . If you say The LORD is my refuge . . . no harm will overtake you . . .

Many have lost their way in the ravaging terrain of pain and depression. But I am with you as you go through this dark valley.

I am the good Shepherd who always looks after my own. And My child, you belong to Me. I am here to retrieve you. I am here to rescue you. I am here to redeem you. Depression is only a shadow threatening you with the idea that your travails have been hopeless. Your pain is another shadow that has convinced you that you are alone, and the pain will never end (Psalms 23 New King James Version)[§].

Do not believe what is in the shadows, because I am there also. My light is what allows the shadows to exist, and it is confirmation that I am with you. Know that My light is greater. I Am greater. Daughter, my great light is in you. Do not allow the shadow to overcome you. The shadow cannot harm you. Stand up and let the light I have given you shine. If you trust me, you will come to know that I have already defeated the darkness that surrounds you. I ask you, my Beloved, what is greater, the object that creates shadow or the light that surrounds it?

I came to myself as His words bore through the throne on which I'd placed my pain. I realized that while I was under attack my emotions had built a temple. I worshiped my despair and made an idol of fear, depression, and pain. Regret came over me. I chastised myself, thinking about God's presence sitting beside me, holding me while I had been weeping hopelessly for months as if He were not there. As if God were not God. Weeping for months as though Jesus's sacrifice meant nothing.

---

§ The LORD is my shepherd; I shall not want. He makes me to lie down in green pastures; He leads me beside the still waters. He restores my soul; He leads me in the paths of righteousness for His name's sake. Yea, though I walk through the valley of the shadow of death, I will fear no evil; For You are with me; Your rod and Your staff, they comfort me. You prepare a table before me in the presence of my enemies; You anoint my head with oil; My cup runs over. Surely goodness and mercy shall follow me all the days of my life; And I will dwell in the house of the LORD Forever.

I'd allowed my pain and uncertainty to dislodge my anchor: His presence. I was heavy with shame for allowing my fears and emotions to be greater than His omnipotent power. I begged for forgiveness.

God's compassionate words caused an overflow in my soul, causing shame and despair to leave the confines of my bound body and imprisoned mind. The power from the Spirit of God that was moving in me began to break the chains of depression. This mass exodus of despondency created space for God's grace to fill me up. It had been months since I felt the presence of God. On this day, I was finally able to feel the embrace of His love.

The majestic sunshine cascading in through the half-opened shutters illuminated the blessings in my life. I realized that despite my physical and mental misery, I also had comfort. My physical capacity, although diminished, was not all gone. I was fortunate to bathe in the sunlight and have a home where all my needs could be met. I had love from Christ, my family, and friends. This sudden awareness of the physical and emotional comfort that was right before me, even in the presence of pain, began to penetrate my hopelessness.

From this moment, I had an epiphany: The darkness I'd experienced for four months could not be the blanket I continued to wrap myself in. Surrounded by His expressions of love, I felt the abundant compassion Christ had for me in my pain. I began to pray and I emerged from this bath differently than I had from my previous baths.

A transformation ignited within my soul; I knew a better solution was on the horizon. A life consumed by pain, pills, and more pain and more pills, and having a sluggish, incapacitated mind and body was a pseudo-life—one I was not intended to live. My back injury and depression pinned me between what my life used to be and what my life was currently—lying in a bed of woefulness with prescriptions forming the pillow for my head. I wasn't sure how to return to my hope-filled life pre-injury, but I knew I couldn't stay pinned.

Although my enemies' pain and depression crept and crawled in the sinews of my mind, slowly devouring me, I would not continue to be an easy prey. Remembering that the Holy Father planned and determined a good outcome for my situation before it began, I repositioned myself for the victory that was secured when I accepted my Heavenly Father's son, Jesus Christ. He recognized me as his daughter and endowed me with His power to defeat my enemies (Romans 8:28, Deuteronomy 20:4 Amplified Bible)**. I stood up, wrestled with my enemies within, and vehemently fought back with the power of God inside of me.

To confront the deception in pain, I scrutinized its tactics and analyzed how it was defeating me in body, mind, and Spirit.

The brain, being the overseer for the normal operation of all body systems and functioning as the communication hub and the mediator of homeostasis in the body, perceives all severe pain as life-threatening. The brain doesn't differentiate chronic pain, which poses no immediate risk to life, from a biological standpoint.

Pain is as a lifesaving alarm that preserves life by signaling danger, such as pain at the onset of a heart attack. Sudden chest pain triggers a complex alarm system wired to our senses, thoughts, emotions, and memory. When the brain's pain alarm is activated, panic, fear, and worry arise—yet these emotions are beneficial. They cause a person to immediately seek lifesaving medical attention.

When the body is in pain, the brain enters into survival mode, which causes emotional stress. The brain's only objective is to stop pain quickly and by any means necessary to maintain life. To accomplish the lifesaving purpose, the brain perceives all pain as internal imbalance

---

** Romans: And we know (with great confidence) that God (who is deeply concerned about us) causes all things to work together (as a plan) for good for those who love God, to those who are called according to His plan and purpose

Deuteronomy: For the LORD your Gord is the one who goes with you to fight for you against your enemies to give you victory

that needs to be corrected. It uses chemical messengers to flood the brain and body with continuous alarm signals. These messengers send and receive messages from brain and the body. They report the internal and external status of body to the brain. This physiological reaction to pain orchestrates our emotional and physical response to eliminate perceived harm. The brain's response to pain is not intended to induce prolonged mental stress, but to get our undivided attention to resolve life-threatening harm.

Life-sustaining stability in the body is primarily maintained by two types of chemical messengers: neurotransmitters and hormones. These messengers not only aid in preserving life but also regulate pleasure and happiness. When stress, anxiety, and fear are in excess it is biologically more difficult to attain enjoyment and depression is highly probable[21].

Sadly, for many with chronic pain, the protective pain response turns against us. The fear and panic useful during acute chest pain becomes destructive because these emotions do not always turn off. Anxiety produces fear, fear induces uncertainty, uncertainty erodes hope, and rational judgment fades. This perpetual cycle takes over rational thought and degrades the dwelling place of thoughts. The side effect of pain's failsafe system to protect the body harms the emotional mind.

To the detriment of mental health, the brain's transactional chemical design to preserve life makes it an enemy to the Spirit and the emotional mind. It is unconcerned with the intangible factors that comprise a satisfied quality of life. Meaningful relationships and self-determination are irrelevant. The brain values only its currency: chemical balance. It always seeks to maintain a pain-free utopia and functioning body systems.

The brain leverages the debilitating power in severe physical and emotional pain to extort our compliance, such as taking as much medication as possible to reduce the pain and avoiding anything that could increase the pain. The emotional mind becomes beholden to fear and anxiety that is deployed by the chemical construct in the brain. This is how pain becomes the relentless enemy within. Its chemical assault on the mind generates constant feelings of distress. Each day these feelings held my thoughts captive. My never-ending grief corrupted my faith, and the coercive lifesaving pain response was killing me spiritually and psychologically.

I questioned myself and God. Would I recover and what would that look like? Would I be able to run again? Continue my career? Take long walks? Climb stairs? Resume my hobbies? What would become of intimacy with my husband? What was God doing while I was hurting? Physical pain weaponized my emotions and infiltrated my peace of mind.

Metaphorically speaking, we have three voices that direct what we do, how we think and feel: the voice from our physical body i.e., arms legs, back, head, etc., and the brain, which regulates pleasure and pain; the voice from our mind, which is the seat of our emotions; and the voice of our Spirit, the part of us that communes with God. Our Spirit is empowered by the Holy Spirit. Because of this, our Spirit has the greatest power and influence compared to the voices from the physical body and the brain. But pain can become the loudest and most influential voice inside of us. When pain screams its demands the noise from a wailing body and mind mutes the Spirit's voice by amplifying physical and emotional despair. When the Spirit is silenced, hope is unprotected, pain besieges faith, and the power of the Spirit is depleted.

Our Spirit has the power to elevate the mind out of depression, pain, and fear. Through the power of faith and the grace of God, the Spirit can override the emotional mind by reconciling our wayward thoughts and emotions with the truth in God's Word. In this way God has endowed our Spirit with complete authority to set our mind at ease. This God-given power of the Spirit makes it our most powerful ally and defender against our adversary's physical and psychological weapons.

Through God's design, the Spirit is not bound by time, place, or circumstance. Simultaneously, it comforts us while removing the fear, anxiety, doubt, and depression that is connected to past encounters and traumatic memories from excruciating pain. It understands the present will always pass and future is underwritten by God's promise. The Spirit remains hopeful of future deliverance regardless of our physical and emotional circumstance. It is always confident, trusts in God, and carries hope, making it the protector of fraughtful mind.

However, because our Spirit resides within our body and mind it is greatly influenced by our emotional and physical state. When we are defeated by insurmountable pain propagated by the brain's chemical pain response, the clamor in the physical body and soul can silence the immutable truths about God's character and His promises to provide peace and wholeness.

Then the distraught mind becomes defenseless against the storms in life. The brain, which is concerned only with preserving its agenda and not how we exist in the world, overpowers our suppressed Spirit. The brain's stress agenda gains complete control, stifles our Spirit, and tosses the emotional mind to-and-fro. Then physical and psychological pain destabilizes our thoughts, which disarms our hope. At this point depression is positioned to take control.

Pain could maintain the upper hand over me if it could keep my mind distracted with the chaos from physical and psychological pain; if uncertainty and loss continued to steal my hope for the future and blind me from the truth in God's promise; if I laid down my Sprit's authority and permitted the arsenal of power within me to remain dormant. But now that I fully understood and could see my enemy, I was positioned to boldly confront and defeat it.

The battleground in my body and mind underwent a tectonic shift, shaking my spiritual and psychological foundation and exposed the fault lines in my faith. Stripped of my ego, I was naked before God. Then He compassionately revealed that my faith had shallow roots intertwined with intellectual beliefs about faith and healing. The fragile roots of my faith needed to be replanted in good soil, free from the thorns of my worries, to grow deeper. He opened my eyes and I was no longer blinded by pain. I saw that I'd taken my faith for granted and my professional confidence was pride in disguise.

My defiance against the enemies within had to come from a place beyond pain's physical and chemical construct. I could not allow pain and depression to dictate my emotional and spiritual response. The only path forward was to repent my character weaknesses, fully embrace my Heavenly Father's Grace, prepare myself to fight with the power of God on my side, and put my faith to work.

CHAPTER SEVEN

Fight

to contend in battle or physical combat;
to defend oneself; to defeat an enemy

Because he was unable to speak, or gesture with his arms, my Dad's attentive gaze was the sign that he recognized me when I said, "Hey Daddy, it's good to see you." Though he towered over me, it was effortless to help him sit up on the edge of the hospital bed and place him in a wheelchair. He was a victim of an array of self-imposed and external tragedies that led to his current circumstance. Seeing my Dad aged well beyond his 48 years shattered my heart. Instead of the 25-year-old woman who understood life's complexities, I became the little girl who yearned for her Dad to be restored to the hero he once was.

It was the Fourth of July, one of his favorite holidays and I wanted to remind him of life beyond the bleak white sterile hospital walls. So

I rolled him outside for him to experience some fresh air, to hear the sounds of nature, and to feel the summer heat we were never bothered by when we gathered for our annual family BBQ.

I chatted endlessly about good memories from our past, hoping he would somehow indicate he understood what I was saying. Surprisingly, his slumped posture began to slowly change. He lifted his head slightly and briefly looked toward the sky. I was glad that for the first time in two months, he noticed the outdoors. But more so, I was grateful I could share this moment with him, in the presence of God, under the sun He created.

About an hour later, I pushed my Dad back to his room. Before I left, I wrapped my arms around him tightly and held on to him a little longer than usual. Kissing him on the cheek, I caressed his face and tucked him into bed. I didn't know this would be the last time we'd sit together in the sun and the last time I would embrace my father.

All these years later, I told myself this would not be my story too. The story where my life ends in my forties as my father's did because like him, I was now running from pain and into the arms of hopelessness. I vowed to no longer succumb to the ruthless enemies within.

I had to fight for my life, my family, and my soul. I did not survive a premature birth and living the first three months of life in a hospital to die here. I didn't survive freak accidents that might have killed me, to die here. I did not survive sexual assault at thirteen to die here, on this battleground of pain and despair. This was not God's plan.

He did not intend for my life to be reduced to depression, prescriptions drugs, or addiction. I saw the pills for what they really were, the smoke and mirrors in the chronic pain process that never make a person whole. I could not continue to chase the pain-free illusion, because it cost more than I was willing to pay. I had to do something audacious: choose to endure more intense physical pain so I could have an alert mind to fight for my spiritual and emotional well-being. I had to stop taking the prescribed pills that were crippling me.

If I continued to rely only on my surgeon's expertise and Dr. P.'s prowess to save me, my life as I knew it would surely end. They'd reached the limits of their skills to aid in my full recovery.

This is not to say the role of spinal injections, anti-inflammatory medications, and nerve pain medications don't have a role in the recovery process for severe back pain—they do, but they're not a comprehensive intervention that results in wholeness when the side effects of physical disability and mental health go unaddressed.

I needed an intervention that could permanently heal my spiritual and psychological pain with a zero percentage of failure. Only divine intervention could defy my constant physical pain and mental torture. I would have to extend my faith farther, deeper, and to a level that could activate what I so desperately needed.

I let go of the hope I gave to my doctors and prescriptions, and I fervently stretched my hand to Jesus Christ. The historical account of the miracles Jesus Christ performed gave me courageous hope to believe in the miracle I needed, one that enabled me to have peace in the presence of excruciating pain.

Placing all my faith and hope in Christ gave me a better chance of escaping my bed of despair. Believing in Christ's ability to fix what was broken in me did not require taking prescriptions or having surgery—what was broken was my faith and Spirit, and there was no pill for that. For my Spirit to heal, I needed to trust God, the Master Physician, enough to endure the pain long enough for a breakthrough and emotional healing to occur. If I could tap into the faith that changes life's outcome, I knew I could survive this injury and misery with my soul intact. I had everything to lose in the hands of qualified medical professionals, but with God, I had everything to gain.

To reclaim my life, I'd have to stop listening to what my pain and depression conditioned me to do—take pills to get relief—and start listening wholeheartedly to God's Word. The only way to win this war with pain was to go through pain. Endurance, perseverance, and determination would all be required to withstand the despair, deceit, and the downfall that laced each pill. Otherwise, I'd be like a leaf in the wind, passively moving from various prescriptions to spinal injections, detached from my true self. I would be allowing pain to overthrow the life I'd known for over 40 years.

I refused to disappear in the life I'd partnered with God to build. I was still there, regardless of how much pain and depression colluded to pursue their agenda instead of God's. My Spirit hadn't vacated my body, it was just buried in the catacombs of pain. I decided I would rather be fully alive with pain than to swallow the deception in my turbulent emotions and bottles of prescriptions.

Flashbacks from the intensity of the nerve pain gripped my thoughts when I contemplated leaving the safety of my daily pills. Then I recalled how I'd assured my patients, saying, "I'm right here supporting you. I won't let you fall. Trust me. Do not be afraid. If you push against me, I will not be able to fully help you sit up or stand because you are working against me. Let me guide you and let's work together."

I heard God say similar words to me. I got comfortable with being uncomfortable and having pain. During my transference of hope from my doctors' plan to God's plan, I trusted the odds of surviving this tug of war for my life were far better with God. My devotion to my doctors' treatment plan was paid by my absence in my life—I was sleepwalking through it, yet still in pain.

It may seem odd to choose physical pain to gain emotional strength, but that's what happened. I stood on His promise and gained my footing. As my patience increased, so did my faith. As my faith increased, so did my mental fortitude, and the doorway to abundant comfort from my Heavenly Father opened.

I had to trust in God's Word by accepting the protection He had reserved to help me. The scripture in Isaiah 41:10 guarantees that my champion, defender, protector, and guide is always with me. I just needed to be reminded of those assurances while fighting for of my life.

Ignoring the deception within my body, I started fighting against doubt and pain. I would not remain a passenger on this "comatose boat" for recovery. I reached toward Jesus for courage, to dislodge pain's parasitic grip on my mind and body. Remembering my baptismal vows, I promised to accept that Jesus is the son of God and died for my sins . . . to love God and obey His commandments . . . to always have faith and honor God . . . to not place anything above the Heavenly Father. I couldn't allow this vow of love and obedience I made over thirty-seven years ago to be so easily broken.

Just as I instructed my patients to first think about moving their paralyzed limbs—because that thought, and then their attempt to actually move their limbs was the beginning of activating their body to begin its recovery—I had to tell myself to do the same. I had to think about moving the paralyzed parts of my mindset, belief system, and hope. I had to activate the peace of God given to me when I gave my vow to Him.

This peace that was gifted to me is the same type of peace Jesus had when he lamented the events of his physical death. He said to God, "May Your will be done." He willingly surrendered His life to unimaginable bodily torture to fulfill His ultimate purpose (Mathew 26: 38-44 and 26:54 NIV). The peace God bestowed upon me would have to be accessed through my surrender as well.

Once I let go of my despair and doubt, the peace that prevails over physical pain and an overwhelmed mind was obtainable. Jesus's peace in

Gethsemane did not run away and hide; it confronted his fear, confronted his emotional pain, and trusted in God's plan. The same courageous peace that defies the body's protective responses which contradicts God's will was available to me. I had to trust that my pain had a purpose, and that enduring peace was within reach.

I began to think about how Jesus Christ would want me to view my physical and emotional paralysis. Christ would want me to consider this injury as fulfilling what has been purposed for my walk with God. He would expect me to reach for the Holy Spirit, the Comforter God sent to abide in me and embrace the comfort that rests in His truth (John 14:16-17 King James Version)*. The promises in the His Word were waiting for me to accept the redemption he offered from physical pain and depression.

Once I inhabited John 14:27 NIV that says, "Peace I leave with you; my peace I give you. I do not give to you as the world gives. Do not let your hearts be troubled and do not be afraid," my trust in God increased. My anxiety about the unknowns in my recovery without taking the prescriptions lessened. I was finally able to take hold of His peace with both hands. I did not let go.

Once I started embracing God's gift of peace and meditated on those scriptures, the Holy Spirit moved the parts of me I could not. I came to know that someday the relief of being unburdened from my nerve endings, from the fear of the unknown, from guilt, from the shame of doubt and depression, would come. I fully embraced a new pain management plan that included only tenacious faith, God's promise, Tylenol, Motrin, and Epsom salt baths.

The spiritual strategy for this battle within began to unfold and my thoughts elevated from depression to hope. I realized that walking with

---

* . . . he shall give you another Comforter, that he may abide with you forever; even the Spirit of truth . . . you know him; for he dwelleth with you and shall be in you.

God meant He was taking me where He wanted me to be. My recovery was delayed so I could recognize that remaining in the terrain of pain with Him as my guide, was the training ground for me to attain what He had purposed for me—to rely on the power of His Word through trust and surrender.

I was praying for God to fix my situation, heal my back, and remove this burden. But what I needed to pray for was strength and patience to endure this pilgrimage and adopt a broader definition of what it meant to be healed. Recovery was not a restored lumbar disc; it was a healed mind and Spirit. If I could remain aware of God's presence as He walked with me, the bulging disc exerting pressure on my nerves wouldn't have the power to apply that same pressure on my mind.

To eliminate the corruptive power my injury had over my Spirit I viewed my pain through the words of Apostle Paul in 2 Corinthians 4:8–9 NIV: "We are hard pressed on every side, but not crushed; perplexed, but not in despair . . . struck down but not destroyed." Regardless of the blows I experienced, I was still breathing, still alive. That meant God continued to orchestrate my life; all was not lost. I could rise up by trusting in God's Word and use it to free me from pain's control.

Once I was mentally free from a common misconception in recovery—that the absence of physical pain represents healing—I was no longer ambushed by the rush of chemicals in my brain shouting: "Get relief now! Take the pills! This is too much to endure. You are putting yourself first by taking the pills. Just lie here and recover." But the truth was, I wasn't recovering—I was actually lying in a tomb designed to look like the healing process.

My daily retreat in floral-scented salt water transformed from an emotional hiding place to a place of true healing. There, God ministered to me. Now each time a tear fell, my hope increased. I knew He didn't wake me each day to be defeated by pain. I was being renewed. It felt better to wield my power of peace, to exercise my faith, and to look for God's expressions of love for me. I could declare to my pain that God was not finished with me yet and accept the full measure of His grace.

I needed to honor God by accepting this life-changing injury with my faith intact. God has never intended any circumstances in life to result in addiction and depression. His intentions are for me to refocus my eyes of faith and recognize His Will working in me. I was supposed to run away from addictive medication and depression and toward God to access the wholeness He gave me when I accepted Him as my Lord, a wholeness encased in the Living Word. All I had to do was trust Him, not the superficial trust that attests God is real. But, the type of trust that is not conditioned on being physically healed.

The course of my recovery changed when I decided that my faith would be greater than the pain, greater than the fear, greater than the despair. I chose to be confident in His Word and through it I would defeat pain without compromising my well-being. As I began to rely on the greatest Healer of all, I concentrated all my effort and energy on God's promise to supply all my needs and to never leave me.

By grace I became strategic in this battle for my mind and soul. Every time I felt "lightning" pass through my body, I prayed—prayer was my defense. The more I hurt, the more leaned into His word and I resisted the overwhelming urge to give in to depression. This regimen of petitioning God, understanding and accepting His word, positioned me to have unwavering belief in God's Word and to be comforted by His bold peace while I was hurting.

When physical pain assaulted me, my faith held me up; it kept me from collapsing. With each painful step, my faith gained more power, and I got mentally stronger. Pain's chemical influence, which caused dread and anxiety to invade my thoughts, occurred with less intensity because it could not fully breach my walls of hope.

I flooded my thoughts with the promises He made: *I will never leave you; I will never put more on you than you can bear; I am your comforter; your healer; and through Me all things are possible.* I needed no prescription to believe in my new treatment plan of choosing brave faith and determination to live an abundant life with His word as my shield.

I accepted the triumph over my pain would not be delivered on my terms. God was not making a shortcut through the wilderness of transformation He was walking me through. On this journey, my spiritual maturity was growing alongside my constant pain. Although the physical conditions for what God was spiritually developing in me was painful, I understood there was not an epidural for the pain that transforms faith.

During this time of spiritual delivery, I held on to God's hand. Kept breathing. Inhale. Exhale. Repeat. I told myself, "Don't be afraid of the trepidation in my thoughts that threatens to take over. Listen to God. Push against those thoughts. Push out fear, despair, sadness, and grief. Push out doubt and give birth to a resurrected Spirit."

I nurtured and strengthened my revived Spirit by activating my faith and fighting through incredibly painful days without my reliable pills. I received tranquility by meditating on God's Word and waited for deliverance without an expectation of when it would happen. Knowing God has determined the end of all "things" enabled me to humble myself as His child and patiently wait on God to reveal what He had already worked out. After all, who was I to rush God in His sovereign process?

I reconciled myself with my adversarial relationship with pain. I couldn't control when my nerves would mount an attack, but I had complete control over my response. I kept my pain on a leash when I activated peace and praise—the essential spiritual weapons that dismantle pain's raid on hope. Pain could roam within my body but not in my thoughts or Spirit.

Pain tried to be the loudest voice in my life and position itself as my dictator. But I could only listen to one voice, one command at a time. I could listen to my pain and depression or to my Lord and Savior. I immersed myself in the living Word of God through praise, worship music, and reading the Bible. The rhythmic notes and verses elevated my thoughts from mourning to high praise. I was thankful my Spirit did what God created it do: listen to Him and minister to me.

I deployed faith that was greater than pain. I prayed constantly and used natural and homeopathic remedies to give my body a hiatus from pain spikes. I courageously called upon the supernatural power that protects all I hold sacred and makes me who I am. I wielded my faith as a weapon, a sword of truth, to strike down the lies my pain and depression were spewing. Each time I swung it, I got stronger.

I also mediated on Romans 8:35, 37–39 NIV: "Who shall separate us from the love of Christ? Shall trouble or famine . . . No in all these things we are more than conquerors through him who loved us. For I am convinced that neither death nor life . . . neither the present nor the future, nor any powers . . . nor anything else in all creation, will be able to separate us from the love of God that is in Christ Jesus our Lord."

This means that nothing, including physical pain, doubt, shame, depression, or guilt, has leverage over my relationship with God or can separate me from His love—which is peace and wholeness. This also meant being a conqueror was already in my DNA. With this revelation I repositioned myself to be the conqueror God had ordained and decided that my physical pain and depression would not overrule my peace of mind. This shift in perspective further empowered my recovery as I continued to decide pain would no longer defeat me.

My power came from integrating God's Word into my conscious thoughts. With Him, recovery was waiting for me to reach it. Knowing my faith could be greater than the nerve endings sending electric volts from my back down to my feet each time I took a step or reached for something, turned over in bed, or sat in a chair, I became single-minded in my hope by keeping my mind on His principles.

I took back the territory of my mind. As my hope increased, so did my faith. I encouraged myself to believe and began to gain more psychological freedom. The victory over my pain wasn't a sudden cessation of pain; it was when my Spirit prevailed. In my Spirit, I knew God was fulfilling his Word in me. I felt His loving presence. I vowed not to let Him down by allowing physical and emotional pain to subdue me. I was able to concede without bitterness or resentment that overcoming pain meant making adjustments in my lifestyle.

Having decided to endure my pain, I was no longer a captive of pain, even when my pain did not decrease. Although my condition was not changing physically, transformation was occurring internally. I considered this stage of my recovery as spiritual germination. While nothing was changing on the surface, underneath the soil of my Spirit, the seeds of hope were developing strong roots of faith. In time, the evidence of faith would sprout and produce fruit of immeasurable joy.

The more I confronted and fought pain like an adversary, the stronger my defense became. The more I believed in my ability to overcome my pain, my Spirit shouted: "God, I trust you! I will not doubt! Strengthen me! I know you have a purpose for me going through this bulging disc storm. Christ is my champion, and I stand on Your Word." I began to have better days. The mental fog from the medication began to lift. Each day I encouraged myself, "By faith I will get through this."

Although I still had pain I was no longer in mental agony over it. I could finally see more of the light that my pain and depression hid from me. I could rest with Jesus holding me. In time, and with much prayer, I rid myself of my recovery timeline and rejected my expectation of living totally pain free. My new expectation of my life with this permanent condition was that I would live with some physical pain, but I would enjoy my life fully. I'd count myself not as a victim, but as a fighter surrounded with the armor of God, fighting negativity daily with bold hope and brazen peace.

Buoyant with God's promise, I felt myself approaching victory. I experienced His peace more than the anxiety from unremitting pain. Each day I told God, "Yes, I still trust you if my physical pain does not end. Yes, I still have hope in the future you promised me." Eventually, my body and mind had intermittent periods of time with less pain that lasted thirty minutes to an hour. Those instances became more frequent and lasted longer. There were some days that I had up to three hours with minimal pain before it became more arduous.

I waited faithfully, tearfully, and in expectation of God's promise materializing in my life. His generous peace coupled with these moments of relief were like a glimmer of sun peeking through my cloud of emotional and physical pain. After five months of fighting for my mind, body, and soul, I prevailed.

CHAPTER EIGHT

Pain

physical and mental suffering or distress
caused by illness, injury or disease

Although my experience with chronic pain is from a back condition, I'd be remiss not to discuss the collective issues associated with disabling chronic pain and other types of pain. The term chronic pain describes conditions that last longer than a standard time period for normal healing from an injury/disease. Chronic pain reoccurs and persists for more than three months[22]. Acute pain, on the other hand, is a sudden or new pain caused by episodic circumstances like a back injury, broken leg, broken arm, or burn. Acute pain is considered temporary, lasting less than three months.

The unavoidable snare in the early onset of chronic pain is that it initially begins as acute pain, as in the case of a back injury. The common treatment for severe acute pain commonly includes a "short-term" low-dose of opioid-based medications or drugs with dependence-forming side effects. Unfortunately this short-term intervention does not provide a reliable long-term solution.

The notion that "short-term" use will prevent dysfunctional dependence is risky, given the emotional and physical volatility in which it's introduced. Persons affected by severe acute pain disease/injury that morphs into chronic pain may also be experiencing other disruptive symptoms like weight loss or gain, sleep deprivation, difficulty concentrating, difficulty organizing their thoughts, fatigue, weakness, decreased libido, and depression, which negatively impact their quality of life. The transition from acute to chronic pain is not an isolated change in a person's health. It is a progressive, evolving disease with numerous implications.

Many people with chronic pain may experience more than one source of pain. For example, a patient with chronic back pain may also have neurological diseases such as migraine, fibromyalgia, or neuropathy. This compounds the severity of the impact on their life. In addition, autoimmune diseases like lupus, multiple sclerosis, rheumatoid arthritis, Sjogren's syndrome, and genetic diseases such as sickle cell can cause chronic pain in the spine (back), neck, hips, knees, shoulders, elbows, hands, feet, and muscles.

Muscle, joint, and neurological pain are the most common forms of chronic non-cancer pain. Musculoskeletal conditions including back, hip, shoulder, or knee pain, are projected to increase due to aging, lifestyle changes, and increased awareness and diagnosis. Although low back pain is common, it's not widely known that it is the leading cause of unplanned early retirement. Further, debilitating chronic pain can lead to a sudden loss of income and even poverty, as well as decreased healthcare access and an increase in health-related expenses from doctor visits, prescriptions, and medical tests (MRIs, CT scans, and X-rays).

Neuropathic pain, also called neurological pain, results from malfunctioning nerves due to damage from a stroke, virus, spinal cord injury, bulging disc, or disease process. Once neuropathic pain develops it does not require an external cause to trigger the pain response. The damaged nerves send random, often frequent pain signals to the brain. This pain is usually described as burning, tingling, "electric shock," numbness, pins and needles, pressure, or a stabbing sensation.

Nociceptive pain arises from an injury causing tissue damage to the skin, muscles, bones, and tendons, such as with broken bones or severe burns. These types of traumatic injuries can also lead to chronic neuropathic pain, should permanent nerve damage or chronic musculoskeletal pain occur.

At a 2018 U.S. Food and Drug Administration Chronic Pain public meeting, people living with this disease frequently described daily unrelenting widespread pain, as well as discomfort in other areas of the body[23]. They feared their chronic pain would worsen over time, preventing them from working, caring for their family and themselves, and carrying out daily chores. They reported experiencing loneliness and isolation due to a loss of meaningful relationships with friends and family because of their extensive time alone managing their pain. Many also carried the burden of stigmatization when their chronic pain was misunderstood[24]. Some were labeled drug seekers or addicts because their prescribed medication was considered unreasonable for "normal" pain—as if this concept actually existed for persons with severe chronic pain.

The effects of chronic pain on overall health are pervasive and wide-ranging, impacting all aspects of a person's life. Society at large and some in the medical community don't understand the difference between opioid dependence and addiction.

Dependence is defined as requiring daily medication to keep a chronic condition in remission or in a state that does not jeopardize other organ systems or bodily functions. For example, people with diabetes are dependent on insulin to maintain normal blood sugar levels, and those with high blood pressure require daily medication to maintain normal blood pressure. People with chronic inflammation due to their disease take steroids to manage an internal inflammatory response. This permits the systems in their body to function properly.

Persons with chronic pain who follow their pain regimen and function well in their daily lives by engaging in meaningful activities with adaptation are not addicts. They have a dependence on their chronic daily medications, which may very well be opiates, to manage their symptoms. This enables them to enjoy a productive, meaningful quality of life[25]. However, the stigma of opioids and addiction means they are often negatively judged by healthcare providers and society. Without the prescribed medications, those able to work reported they would be unable to do their jobs. Others stated they would not be capable of getting out bed or to walk[26].

According to the fifth edition of the *Diagnostic and Statistical Manual of Mental Disorders*, addiction is a compulsive physical and psychological need for, and use of a habit-forming substance (heroin, opioids, nicotine, or alcohol) characterized by tolerance and by well-defined physiological symptoms upon withdrawal[27]. Broadly, it is the persistent, compulsive use of a substance known to be physically, psychologically, or socially harmful. Addiction is difficult to overcome due to the chemical euphoria the substance delivers. These substances cause structural and functional changes in the brain's reward, inhibitory, and emotional circuits[28]. As the body's physical and emotional wellness intertwine with addictive substances the brain begins to identify the substance as a necessity to maintain its chemical balance.

There has been a movement in the medical field to address the social stigma surrounding addiction, by using person-first language to remove the negative connotation associated with drug and substance abuse disorders. The term "substance use disorder" (SUD) and "opioid use disorder" (OUD) remove the words that define a person by their condition.

I call SUD and OUD dysfunctional dependence because the continued use an addictive substance persists regardless of the negative impacts on a person's well-being. Self-preservation—maintaining shelter, relationships, a job, or a health concern—are not a priority due to intense craving, obsessive thinking, loss of inhibitory control, and compulsive substance abuse.

Not everyone with chronic pain who takes opioids develops an opioid use disorder, and not everyone with a substance or opioid use disorder experiences chronic physical pain—yet both may experience chronic psychological pain. With depression and anxiety lurking, ready to consume life, OUD and SUD can become bedfellows in the fight against chronic pain.

Pain occurs first in the nervous system; the body part is the recipient. The nervous system is a complex construct of nerves, neurons, synapses, and chemical messengers such as hormones and neurotransmitters that regulate and modulate pain. The sensory infrastructure to detect pain is multifaceted and vast. The pain network is located in the skin, eyes, organs, the body hair, between the joints of bones, and the spinal cord itself. When pain is triggered, a chemical reaction in the body activates signals that cause the sensation of pain.

The pain process in the nervous system functions like an electrical system that produces light with the flip of a light switch. When a wall switch is flipped up, lights automatically come on because the home wiring is connected to a main power source.

Similarly, pain is triggered when an "external switch"—a physical injury or disease process—is activated. Once this switch is flipped "on," the sensation of pain is instant. The pain signal automatically travels to the brain, the body's main power source. The nervous system's network of chemical and physical receptors mediates the conscious experience of pain.

Although the sensation is triggered in various parts of the body, the awareness of pain occurs only in the brain. A person in a coma or sedated by anesthesia does not perceive pain because they're unconscious. An alert brain deciphers the pain message from the body and tells it how to respond, sending an urgent message for the body to "turn off" the switch and stop the pain. Unfortunately, in a person with chronic pain, the on and off switches can malfunction. As a result, their nervous system sends an erroneous signal that physical danger is imminent. This triggers overwhelming worry, anxiety, and fear.

Receptors in the nervous system act as bridges for chemical signals to communicate between the brain and body. Without our control or conscious input, these receptors detect external pressure: vibration, gravity, light, hot, cold, blood pressure, chemicals such as carbon dioxide. They are hardwired throughout our body and organs to regulate all bodily functions, including breathing, heart rate, body temperature, and thirst. These receptors independently relay messages to and from the and brain to preserve life and protect the body from harm[29].

For example, the buildup of carbon dioxide in our blood triggers the automatic protective response for a person to inhale and exhale based on the amount of oxygen the body senses it needs.

The body is designed to protect itself from internal and external threats. The pain response is integrated with receptors to work with our senses: sight, hearing, smell, taste, and touch, so we can perceive danger and respond. For example, our sensory response is what causes us to run out of a burning building when we smell smoke and see fire.

In addition to the five senses, the body activates another proactive mechanism, our memory. The body stores entrenched memories from painful or frightening experiences, so an individual will respond more urgently to protect themselves. When we experience physical or emotional pain such as anxiety or fear, our brain stores the source of that pain as a "trigger," so we can quickly recall and avoid that situation again.

This emotional reaction stored in our memories is how adolescents and adults know that a stove burner is hot and can hurt you. We've been taught about the dangers of fire or had a personal experience with it. Therefore, the brain recalls, and the body responds to these stored memories of fear and danger. If we smell something burning, see black smoke, hear a smoke alarm or feel a surge of heat, we know to leave the area quickly. Our past experiences with and knowledge of fire inform our present-day responses.

The emotional reaction to severe chronic pain is stored in our memories the same way. Our experience with severe pain activates a specific emotional response, including fear, worry, anxiety, and hopelessness. These emotions escalate our pain, like pouring gasoline on a fire. For those with chronic pain, these emotions may never go away. A person with chronic pain is threatened by a metaphorical scorching fire—and is burned by the pain daily. Their actual pain and their memory of pain permanently influences how they engage in their lives[30].

Imagine the threat of a flame engulfing your foot with each step you take, your shoulders and back whenever you reach for a glass of water, your leg whenever you stand up or sit down, your head whenever you turn it or open your eyes? Reflexively self preservation would cause you to avoid this metaphorical fire.

The withdrawal reflexes of someone living with this threat are continually activated. They avoid any situation that can trigger their pain and often overreact to the slightest threat of pain, afraid of what they'll endure. Over time, chronic pain can alter how the nervous system perceives pain. It can become hypersensitive—causing receptors to fire easily and release the chemical reaction that signals pain.

The overactive nervous system causes pain to be more frequent, more intense, or both.

The receptors are the "five-star general" that determines what we should or should not respond to or perceive as a threat. Receptors like the brain are concerned only with homeostasis in the body systems, not hope or faith. They serve our body on the level of pleasure, pain, chemical balance, and the here and now.

The body, that is, the brain's agenda, is achieved at the juncture of our receptors; it is there that physical pain and disillusionment convene. The stage is set to breed depression and additional mental health issues. The body's agenda becomes physical and emotional relief at any cost. This is where addiction hides—in the brain's self-seeking pursuit of pleasure and to be pain free. When the mind and the body experience the defeat of unfulfilled pain relief, a downward spiral of unmet expectations ensues, and emotional malfunction and dysfunctional substance dependency are born.

At its core, pain is the body's security system, deployed to protect us from harm and preserve life. It is not intended to inflict suffering per se, but to sound an internal alarm so we will act to prevent bodily harm.

Pain is a siren that tells us something is wrong. The greater the perceived threat from pain, the louder the alarm will sound, and the greater the intensity of pain experienced. Because the nervous system powers all bodily systems, the brain perceives nerve pain as the greatest threat to life and produces the most intense pain a person can experience. The brain releases an immense physiological arsenal of hormones and other chemicals that trigger internal metabolic stress responses, like anxiety and fear, that compel us to take action.

When acute pain sours into chronic pain, our receptors have strategically stored the pain memory in multiple areas of our brain. This process is the learned pain experience. A person's past experience with pain influences their response when their pain worsens, or they do something that triggers the pain. It is for this reason, a person becomes conditioned to rely on prescriptions and avoid doing activities that have previously exacerbated their pain.

Someone with chronic pain becomes hyper-focused on the pain medication because their mind is occupied with protecting the body from harm. This cycle of constant pain and the fear perpetuates depression, anxiety, and sadly, addiction. Our thoughts, which are influenced by our emotions and past experiences, govern our relationship with pain. The habitual method for coping with severe pain center around pain medication. Not because it's a complete remedy—but because it provides the fastest form of relief. Regrettably, over time, the body and brain become conditioned to pursue pills first.

Once an individual begins to exclusively rely on prescriptions for pain relief, it becomes difficult to step away, even when the pills negatively affect their quality of life. It becomes almost impossible to consider alternatives when doctors, the trusted guides, provide only prescriptions and surgery for the injured body, and no intervention for the injured mind.

The knowledge that chronic pain caused by nerve damage is a blaring, blood-curdling internal alarm is paramount in the fight against chronic pain. Understanding the pain response is our mind's most effective protective mechanism to inform our psychological response.

Because addiction is never the plan, don't allow its stigma to cause even more shame in the person you encounter or hasten the toxic judgment inherent in all stigmas. You never know exactly what happened prior to someone's fall into cycles of dysfunctional dependency. You never know the extent of relief and healing they were looking for when they began to take the prescribed drugs or the pain they may have been running from.

CHAPTER NINE

Errors and Solutions

mistakes and resolutions
for difficult circumstances

My back injury exemplifies how the medical approach typically unfolds. After seeing my general practitioner for acute back pain that did not respond to the standard treatment of short-term muscle relaxers and NSAIDs (non-steroidal anti-inflammatory drugs, i.e., naproxen and ibuprofen). I was referred to a specialist, the neurosurgeon. A person with chronic pain is usually referred to a doctor who specializes in the body system affected by the pain. For instance, an orthopedic surgeon for hip, knee, and shoulder joints; a neurosurgeon for the back or spine; a neurologist for nervous system-related pain like migraine; a rheumatologist for autoimmune-related pain.

The next step is to have imaging—an MRI, CT scan, or X-ray—of the area causing the pain—and possibly blood tests. Once a diagnosis is finalized and the specialist determines the pain is too severe to manage with a short, seven-to-ten day prescription of opioids, a referral to a pain management specialist is made. Due to the prescription drug epidemic, many doctors do not prescribe opioids long-term. A referral to a pain management specialist is seen as the best and only logical solution outside of surgery and a round of physical therapy.

The traditional medical approach for treating chronic pain from a bodily injury or disease is riddled with perilous oversights. They include failure to address the psychological and social impact of the condition at the onset of the diagnosis, establish realistic expectations for recovery, and deficient patient education on the pain process.

These omissions have far-reaching consequences for those with chronic pain and their families. One lapse in any area mentioned above leaves an individual defenseless in the fight for their quality of life. The transition from an acute pain injury or disease process to chronic pain must be handled with more cautionary measures.

The treatment plan from my physicians did not address the psychological impacts of my injury. This oversight contributed to my mental health crisis. It's standard when treating a patient with antiepileptic drugs (also known as anti-seizure drugs) to monitor them for the emergence or worsening symptoms of depression, unusual changes in mood or behavior, and suicidal ideation. But my doctors never conducted a mood screen for the side effects of Gabapentin and Lyrica, both known to increase the risk of suicidal thoughts or behavior.

I was unaware of these life-altering side effects at the time, nor did my doctors disclose this information. They never asked how I was coping or to let them know if my mood and behavior had changed. It is possible the minimized voice that my pain permitted me to have was too small, too quiet, too encrypted for them to hear my cry for help when I said, "I am having a difficult time adjusting to what has happened to me." They replied, "Hang in there." They relegated my state of mind to a normal response to my injury. Although my physicians were some of the best in their fields, they lacked the holistic treatment approach all doctors should provide. They saw only my injury, not me.

Their collective response was a continued discussion about medications and they did not inquire further about my mental health. Like many others going through a health crisis, I was in an emotionally vulnerable state, following the lead of physicians—not advocating for emotional support. As a result, my mental health suffered.

Due to the severity of chronic pain and its associated disability, opioid analgesics are now the most prescribed class of medications in the U.S., regarded as being the most effective at suppressing pain[31]. However, when psychological injury is not addressed with the same robust efforts as physical pain, opioid analgesics have a higher risk of severe repercussions.

According to the National Institute on Drug Abuse (NIDA), in 2022 a minimum of 41 people people died each day from prescription related opioid overdoses, totaling 14,716 deaths.[32] This is more than heroine-related overdoses at 5,871, cocaine overdoses at 5,868, and benzodiazepines (Xanax, Valium, Ativan) at 10,964[33]. Which means controlled legal prescription drugs are not necessarily less harmful than illegal drugs.

The failure to manage the full scope of chronic pain has resulted in significant morbidity (illness) and mortality (death) independent of sociodemographic factors. Research shows the lifetime prevalence for chronic pain patients attempting suicide is between 5% and 14% and their thoughts of suicide are approximately 20%[34,35].

What happens to parents who can no longer provide for their families on a disability income or when depression wrecks their lives? What about the person who lacks a support system and is now unable to support themselves, financially or emotionally? These questions and other social determents of health deserve the utmost attention in addressing the chronic pain epidemic.

Medical professionals are aware of the interdependent relationship between pain and mental health. Physicians, as experts in preserving life and fostering healing and recovery, are entrusted by patients to protect and guide them. People expect advice on the short- and long-term impacts of their conditions and to be referred to the appropriate medical specialists. But initial treatment plans often focus only on the acute, short-term impairment in the body and neglect a long-term plan to handle chronic pain's lifelong pysychosocial impact.

When the medical community prioritizes pain over the patient experiencing the pain, it removes the holistic approach to care and neglects how the person's physical condition impacts all areas of their life—relationships, careers, hobbies, and mental health.

Many physicians don't ask about their patients' emotional responses to pain, unintentionally neglecting to address the underlying causes that contribute to SUDs and OUDs. This failure may stem from time constraints on patient visits, which, sadly, is pervasive today. Or perhaps the question has not occurred to the physician. Or perhaps it has, but they are ill-equipped to respond. Regardless, inadequate attention to coping strategies and inadequate emotional support compounds mental and psychosocial stressors following a new diagnosis.

Having personally experienced the transition from acute pain to chronic pain it became obvious that the transition begins when the initial diagnosis of an injury or disease process that is known to lead to chronic pain disease is confirmed. This perilous transition should not begin twelve weeks after the diagnosis is made.

By the time a doctor has waited three months to confirm the anticipated chronic pain diagnosis, the ill-informed individual has been succumbing to their pain's side effects. Unmet expectations and disappointment become fuel for dysfunctional coping.

The consequences are catastrophic when few efforts are made during this twelve week delay to mentally prepare individuals for the significant life-changing event that occurs at the onset of a chronic pain diagnosis. Individuals with chronic pain are likely to have significantly higher rates of alcohol consumption, smoking, obesity, and OUD and SUD. They also have an increased risk emotional disturbance because the physiological process for pain and emotions relies on some of the same neurotransmitters for regulating mood and they can become dysregulated[36,37].

The prevalence of chronic pain and its inextricable correlation with mental health strongly imply that a comprehensive effort should be made to prioritize psychosocial support at the onset of the treatment plan. With the mortality rate of those with chronic pain being two times higher than that of the general population, the approach I suggest would be equivalent to the standard proactive methods for prevention in other high mortality diseases like diabetes, heart disease, and high blood pressure[38].

Early health risk screening, patient education, and referrals to other supportive medical professionals are paramount to prevent the complications for those diseases, which can quickly become life-threatening when not carefully managed. Likewise, individuals with chronic pain that is not managed carefully are also at risk for life threatening complications. I believe if the medical community broadened the chronic pain treatment approach to also include preserving mental health it could address the gap filled by maladaptive coping habits.

To promote well-being and establish assimilation of a new medical condition, individuals with heart disease, diabetes, and high blood pressure are taught at the onset of their diagnosis to adapt to the disease process by modifying their diets and lifestyle. Similarly, adaptation and acceptance, along with modification, remains key for individuals with chronic pain to have a better quality of life as well[39]. Establishing realistic expectations for chronic pain conditions is essential to mitigate the deleterious side effects. However, the primary way physicians manage individuals with chronic pain who fail to adapt is to limit the dosages and frequency of prescribing medications instead of addressing the underlying issues[40].

Doctors should consider a person's ability to engage in their home life, their relationships, physically care for themselves, and their ability to return to work. A holistic intervention implemented at the onset of the recovery process would meet these physical and psychosocial needs.

I suggest that after four weeks when disabling acute pain is likely to become chronic pain, the primary care physician leading the treatment plan should make referrals not only to the physical therapist to rehabilitate the physical body but also to a psychologist and an occupational therapist—those better qualified to address issues pertaining to adaptation, modification, integration, and acceptance of sudden lifestyle changes. The occupational therapist and psychologist are knowledgeable about training, educating, and empowering patients to adapt to physical disability and chronic pain and how to prevent flawed emotional responses and thought processes.

Someone with sudden pain that prevents them carrying out everyday tasks can be devastated, especially when the ETA on their recovery has passed the expected timeframe. Without early intervention, patients with chronic pain lose both physically and psychologically. Establishing realistic expectations for chronic pain disorders and disease is essential to help maintain an individual's quality of life.

Mental health professionals play a crucial role in helping people deal with the psychological challenges of chronic pain. Psychologists, with their training in the social, medical, and emotional aspects of chronic pain, are proficient at addressing the complex relationship between emotions, behaviors, and opioid use. They provide a nonjudgmental, supportive atmosphere, along with structure and accountability that helps patients understand and respond to the effects of pain on their choices, thoughts, and behavior.

Additionally, their expertise in diagnosing and treating mental health issues a patient may or may not be aware of can help address any underlying medical history that can complicate a patient's response to their injury or disease.

Occupational therapists' specialized training integrates medical models of disease processes, illness, injury, neurology, psychology, and sociology. In rehabilitation, their approach and expertise can be seen as a hybrid between that of a physical therapist and a psychologist. Their focus is on a person's ability to physically perform the activities of daily living as well as their emotional and cognitive ability to meaningfully meet those desired obligations that are essential to their quality of life.

Occupational therapists take a holistic approach to facilitating recovery, examining multiple levels of dysfunction and disability. The first level is physical: How a person's eyes, ears, arms, hands, and legs function. The second level is neurological: How the nervous system and brain function in the body. The third level is psychosocial: How an individual's mental health influences their views and social life. That is, how a patient views themselves internally. Do they see themselves as confident and capable? How do they believe others view them? The last level is cognitive: How well can individual utilize coping and adaptation strategies? This level addresses reasoning, judgment, and memory capacity.

Occupational therapists meticulously analyze all barriers that can impede someone's daily physical and emotional performance. They identify and remediate limited strength, joint mobility, balance, coordination, neurological impairments, and in pain. They also address anxiety, memory issues, depression, and psychosis, through adaptation and compensatory strategies to help individuals maintain functional engagement in their daily life.

To enable a patient with an impairment to carry out their daily activities, occupational therapists assess how the person can modify and adjust their external environments—in the bedroom, bathroom, kitchen, laundry room, office, or other workplace, and the interior of their vehicle—to accommodate their disability. They also teach patients how to adapt physically and emotionally to those changes.

Anyone with chronic pain faces challenges that require more than intuition to endure. No one is born knowing how to overcome physical and psychological pain on our own. We all need help to handle the grief and loss that accompanies long-lasting severe pain and the resulting disability that can follow. A sudden change in a person's health impacts the physical aspects of their life and can cause an invisible emotional injury as well.

As an occupational therapist, I knew the physical modifications I could make to avoid exacerbating my pain and meet my basic daily needs—getting out of bed, walking, getting in the tub, dressing myself, etc. In that way, I had an advantage. But even with my mental health training, during my emotional collapse I could not access the full scope of my professional skills to avoid the psychological stress of ceaseless pain.

I would have benefited from a referral to a mental health professional early on in the treatment plan. We could have discussed my plans to cope and identified any emotional blind spots. I could have developed a proactive strategy to deal with the potential emotions that arise with prolonged pain, such as anger, grief, and depression. It would have been helpful to have someone I could confide in about my most terrifying and embarrassing thoughts that I couldn't bring myself to share out loud with those who love me most.

Meeting the complete physical and psychological needs of those contending with chronic pain requires intervention at the acute pain stage of the injury, disorder, or disease. The expertise of a psychologist and occupational therapist is most beneficial for those at risk for chronic pain at the onset of the acute diagnosis already causing them to adjust and modify how they live their lives. With timely intervention by these mental health professionals, the chronic pain population will have a better chance of attaining a more fulfilling quality of life[41].

The next, and perhaps the most important part of a proactive treatment approach is teaching individuals about the pain response. Teaching people how the body detects pain and why it reacts as it does can demystify chronic pain by reducing it to its lowest common denominator: a multitude of signals from the nervous system. Separating fact from fiction about pain is key to equipping patients with a fighting chance to preserve their quality of life. This vital information is foundational in helping an individual with chronic pain to persevere.

I recall that blunt nauseating feeling of powerlessness over the spasms, the frequent random stabbing pains, and feeling like the lower half of my body was being electrocuted. I had no control over the grief and anger that suffocated me daily—or the sadness that greeted me each morning and tucked me in bed each night. I didn't choose to have excruciating, debilitating pain and its accompanying depression, nor do others in the chronic pain community. They want to feel better and be who they once were, but often, pain exerts total control. Then, they begin to withdraw from their life in the mistaken belief that withdrawal is their sole means of survival.

The chronic pain agenda is complicated because the emotional response is based upon facts and our less true catastrophized emotions.

It's a fact that a person with chronic pain may not be able perform the physical tasks they once did. The sadness and loss experienced is real, due to the abrupt changes in their life. It may also be true that they must reconsider and restructure their career.

But what's false is that unbearable pain must drive a person to a reduced standard of living and submit to a life dictated by chronic pain. It's by no means easy to confront an overbearing nervous system, but with intentionality, it's possible for an individual to carve out aspects of themselves that they prohibit pain from altering.

I did not initially realize I was going through the five stages of grief described in my college textbooks. The countless lectures and practicums never crossed my mind as I wavered between denial, anger, bargaining, and depression. The last stage, acceptance, evaded me for months. Depression roamed unimpeded by the gatekeepers I passively deferred to for my recovery. The emotional undercurrent of severe pain was drowning me. My physicians response to my SOS was to say, "Slow down. This can be difficult."

Inadvertently, my physicians put me on a path that required me to tend to my own mental health. My doctors failed to offer an appropriate referral, and I failed to ask for one. The words I so often used to advocate for the mental health of others was buried under my depression and shame. But I was fortunate to be able to rely on my spiritual foundation and aspects of my professional training.

Hopefully, if you or someone you know encounters chronic pain, they will meet medical professionals who set realistic expectations for chronic pain management—ones not focused on a cure or a complete pain-free outcome. Effective pain management should concentrate on positive lifestyle changes through modification and adaptation. This new way of life does not mean avoiding living a full, productive life; rather, it involves engaging in an alternative lifestyle.

For individuals to achieve a positive adjustment to a life with chronic pain, they need help to navigate domains of life such as work and home life, physical and emotional well-being, and relationships. The colossal task of maintaining a life shattered by chronic pain and disability requires more than just the neurosurgeon, pain management doctor, neurologist, or rheumatologist; it requires a psychologist, occupational therapist, support system, and possibly homeopathic practitioners.

CHAPTER TEN

Return to Work

coming back to do the job

Returning to work meant the beginning of my public walk of faith. The confidence I'd been practicing privately with God would be on public display.

Thinking about my return to work, I questioned whether I could duplicate the unbreakable faith I'd had in the presence of God in my home, my private sanctuary. Would my fear of reinjuring myself overwhelm me? Would my uneasiness about how my body would feel after a workday become Worry 2.0? Would the threat of pain uproot my recently planted seeds of faith, hope, and trust when my nerves constricted in my back?

I couldn't ignore the nervousness that surfaced from the thought of holding on to my faith at the accelerated pace of a workday compared to the unhurried tranquil hours spending time with God's Word ministering to my soul. Sorting through the wreckage from my injury, I faced my anxious thoughts and took the lessons I'd learned with me to work. I'd need to keep them as close as the breath I breathe.

I held tightly to the significance and power of God's presence. I learned that if I stayed completely aware in mind and Spirit of the greatness of His presence, and immersed myself in that truth, there was no gap He could not fill. The emptiness my anxiety and the fear of the unknown created would be eliminated. If I stayed tethered to His presence, the gap between having no bulging disc and thriving with a bulging disc did not exist: His presence filled the gap.

As I inhaled oxygen, the perfect mixture of atmospheric elements He created to sustain life, I was acutely aware of God's presence in every breath. His presence was in the innermost parts of my body that he designed to preserve my life. It was in my lungs that He created to effortlessly inhale and exhale and in my heart that He created to automatically beat. If I truly believed that I'm His treasured creation, I would never again be shaken by "what ifs" as I transitioned back to work.

I was empowered by the knowledge that my body is the same flesh and bone that Jesus walked in during his ministry on Earth. Christ modeled that the body is a tool used to fulfill God's plan for us. My body is still here and functioning, still purposed to occupy the positions in my life as wife, mother, daughter, sister, friend, therapist, and a child of God. It can still be used to fulfill His purpose. I would never lie in the bed of depression and fear again. I'd burned the bed I'd laid in for five months and discarded its ashes, along with my professional and spiritual arrogance. My faith was renewed and resurrected to fulfill God's intention for the life He gifted me.

Another lesson I carried with me was the importance of relying on the character of God. If I could remain cognizant that His love is merciful when He corrects me, expands my faith, and reveals more of Himself to me, I would always be comforted during episodic periods of pain. God testing my faith during my injury was not punishment or a reprimand. It was a trial for me to become who He intended me to be, a true representation of His grace, His peace, and His word.

The next lesson I retained was the principality precept. A principality is an entity that rules a particular region. Pain and depression are principalities positioned to rule in our body and mind. Together they leverage physical and emotional pain (fear, anxiety, loss, anger, and doubt) to subjugate us to their authority. They disarm our psychological armor by destroying the spiritual fruits of joy, peace, patience, faithfulness, and self-control. These principalities lurk and look for who they can devour (1 Peter 5:8–9 NIV)*.

I fought the pain and depression principalities for my Spirit to rule the territory of my mind. Because of this journey with God, I was prepared for the tactics of my enemies within. I was able to shield my thoughts, stand firm on my faith and the truth in His word about hardship and abide in His strength and power (Ephesians 6:10–17 NIV)†.

I carried with me the revelation that God trusts us with many forms of trials and tribulations, such as loss of loved ones, changes in health, and traumatic circumstances. Being a child of God means that at some point in our life we will encounter a Job-like season and should adopt his faithful response: "Though He slay me, yet will I trust Him . . ." (Job 13:15 NIV). Even when my pain threatened my peace and hope, I reclaimed my faith. By grace, I saw my pain for it what it was—an overactive nervous system sending me false signals that my life was over. I held His banner of restoration high, with strong arms of truth and legs

---

* Be alert and of sober mind. Your enemy . . . prowls around like a roaring lion looking for someone to devour. Resist . . . standing firm in the faith.

† Be strong in the Lord and in his might power. Put on the full armor of God, so that you can take your stand . . . for our struggle is not against flesh and blood . . . but against the powers of this dark world . . . take up the shield of faith . . . and the helmet of salvation . . .

of faith to support me. I carried His light and His promise with me to work, and I clothed myself with His grace daily.

I also carried with me the lesson from my relationship with God as it transitioned from Savior, Protector, Provider, and Friend to Lord. I knew God as my Savior because He rescued me from the precipice of disabling depression. I came to know Him better as a Protector when he shielded me from the destruction of despair. I saw Him more clearly as my Provider when he gave me the revelation that He was still providing for me, and all was not lost. We grew closer as Friends when I took my eyes off Him and covered my ears with my sorrow. Instead of judgment He extended mercy. He told me, "I am the Lord of mercy. My mercy and compassion are renewed every morning. I am faithful and My compassion does not fail" (Lamentations 3:22–23 NKJV).

During this battle for my soul, I came to know God intimately as my Lord—not in the formal sense of His dominion over what occurs in my life, but as the Lord I serve. Because He is my Lord, I willingly submit myself to His divine purpose and plan even when I am hurting. His priorities become mine and I relinquish my plans for His. My duty in honoring my Lord is to follow His plan for my life, regardless of the challenges, including the painful, restricted state of my body. As Jesus's representative, I could not carry both the weight of my anxiety and the light of His deliverance. Each day I had to choose to keep the door closed on the darkness of insecurity and allow His eternal light to shine in me (John 8:12NIV)‡.

Because I chose to surrender and wear His grace, God recognized my humble Spirit and ministered to me. The Holy Spirit, the Comforter, the Advocate, the Counselor, the Strengthener, the Standby continually reminded me of everything He said to me and of His love for me

---

‡ I am the light of the world. Whoever follows me will never walk in darkness but will have the light of life.

(John 14:25-26 AMP). As I abided in Him during my transition back to work, the Holy Spirit shielded me from the doubt and apprehension attempting to undermine my faith and trust in Him.

I replayed in my mind a conversation God had with me during one of our many bathtub encounters. He said,

My Daughter, you can get through this.

You can find Me because I am right there with you.

Open your eyes to see Me.

Take off the blindfold of pain and depression and fear.

I have spoken all things into existence and now I speak peace in

and to your circumstance.

I speak wholeness in all the places this pain has broken you.

I spoke to your pain and I, the Alpha and Omega, have the victory because

your soul and your Spirit reside in My everlasting Kingdom.

I command you, My Daughter, to live through My Word and

I will always be the lamp at your feet guiding you.

I am the shepherd that goes before you and makes your crooked paths straight.

I have ordained your destiny, and this fear and defeat is not where you live.

Walk with Me and I will show you the way.

I did as He commanded. I walked with Him and I prepared for my first day back at work. After six months the spasms were significantly less intense, and my back pain was manageable with over-the-counter medications and aquatic therapy. To limit physical stress on the muscles in my back, I enlisted the help of my son and husband to do the heavy chores around the house, such as mopping and vacuuming, which require repetitive bending. I resumed preparing my family's favorite meals, with some modifications to my dinner preparation routine, and I was enjoying nature again with short walks to the park.

At first it was strange returning to my desk and seeing the schedule dated in the fall of the previous year. It was a reminder of how much time had truly passed. The trees and shrubs outside my office window were in full bloom; the crape myrtles showed signs that summer was near.

I meditated on God's timing and seasons and the scripture in Ecclesiastes 3:1–8 NIV came to mind: ". . . a time to plant and a time to uproot . . . a time to tear down and time to build, a time to weep and a time to laugh, a time to mourn and a time to dance . . ." My weeping and mourning seasons had ended, and the time of my pruning was over. It was time to be fruitful again by returning to do the work that I committed to doing and help those in need of rehabilitation to adapt to their sudden changes in their physical and cognitive ability.

Returning to work meant I'd need to make some modifications to how I did the physical aspects of my job. Thankfully, my career prepared me to adjust to my new normal. Instead of relying on physical strength, I used a height-adjustable hospital bed to assist patients into a standing position and I relied on mechanical lift equipment to help someone move from a bed to a wheelchair.

My expertise in ergonomic workspace adaptation and modification was even more useful than before. Ergonomics is the applied science of designing and arranging tools, equipment, and workspaces to promote efficiency and prevent overuse injuries. An ergonomic workstation supports the body's natural position and alignment while seated or standing when using job-related tools or equipment. For instance, a person who spends hours working on a computer should have height-adjustable, pivotable, and tilting features for their computer screen, chair, and desk to avoid straining the muscles and ligaments their neck, shoulders, and wrist while working.

So before returning to work I asked for an ergonomically correct chair that featured a height-adjustable seat and armrest, adjustable lumbar support, and reclining back support. I could no longer sit in a basic office chair or a rolling stool for hours to complete the required computer tasks.

To prevent my own reinjury, I implemented a form of "Back Protection Strategies" I'd taught my patients recovering from back surgery. I continued core strengthening exercises, avoided twisting and rotating my back, and I never lifted or carried items greater than twenty pounds. I used a rolling cart to avoid pulling or carrying heavy equipment from one side of the building to the other. I also frequently sat down after 30 minutes of standing, to incorporate intermittent rest which is recommended to prevent overuse injuries in the work place.

At the end of my first day back at work, I thought about the thousands of others like me—people with chronic pain who have taken extensive time away from their jobs and fought hard to return to work. I realized it's a journey no one is prepared for. The uncharted realm of physical rehabilitation, the short-term disability process, and the Family Medical Leave Act (FMLA) process to secure a person's job can be stressful. Few in the medical field or people's employers consider the financial burden someone with severe pain must carry. I was glad I elected to purchase the employer-offered short-term disability coverage. Although the weekly checks I received were just a percentage of my regular pay, the funds were very beneficial. However, access to short-term disability is not always an option due to cost, or an employer not offering it.

I was fortunate to be able to pay the additional fees for my doctor to complete short-term disability paperwork updates every three weeks, the biweekly copays for both of my doctors, and to withstand the loss of income. For many, that is not possible. Many people turn to government financial assistance or to family and friends to cover routine expenses like rent, medical insurance, utilities, car and life insurance, and groceries—all because of a sudden disability from intractable pain.

I've prepared a list of questions to ask a doctor and employer in the process of navigating an acute medical condition that could lead to a chronic condition and extended leave of absence from work.

Questions for Your Doctor

1. What are all the side effects of the medication you are prescribing?

2. Is depression or a change in mood a possible side effect?

3. What is your plan for me to address mental health changes if they arise?

4. Do you have a psychologist or licensed counselor you can refer me to?

5. Which of the doctors coordinating my recovery is responsible for completing disability and FMLA forms? Will it be the neurosurgeon, neurologist, orthopedic physician, referring primary doctor, or pain management specialist?

6. Will there be a charge each time you complete a disability update to recertify that I am unable to return to work?

7. Due to the physical limitations caused by my injury or disease, will I have a chronic condition requiring lifetime management that could result in a permanent disability?

8. Based upon my job description, will I require accommodations to return to work?

9. Which doctor will complete my employer forms to notify them about the medically necessary accommodations I need to return to work?

10. Will the recommendations from the physical and occupational therapist be considered when you deem my condition medically stable enough for me to return to work?

Questions for Your Employer

1. What is the FMLA process?

2. Are there additional guidelines the company adheres to for me to return to work?

3. Can you provide me with a detailed job description that includes the physical requirements for my job?

4. What options are available for me to pay for my medical insurance while I am on leave from work?

5. Will you implement the accommodations my physician deems medically necessary for me to return to work?

6. How long will it take to implement those accommodations?

If you require accommodations to perform your job, review the required duties in your job description prior to returning to work. The Americans with Disability Act (ADA) of 1990 provides some protection for people with documented disabilities. To qualify for ADA protections, you must have a documented impairment that significantly limits or restricts a major life activity such as hearing, speaking, performing manual tasks, walking, or caring for oneself.

The ADA also states that reasonable accommodations may include modifying equipment, job restructuring, a part-time or modified work schedule, modifying training materials, providing readers and interpreters, and making the workplace readily accessible to and usable for people with disabilities. It is also a violation of the ADA to fail to provide reasonable accommodation to those with known physical and mental limitations unless doing so would impose an undue financial or structural burden to the company. Many companies have a Human Resource department available to provide specific information about your employer's disability policies.

CHAPTER ELEVEN

Depression

a low place; pressed down

I have always had an abundance of patience, kindness, and compassion for those with depression. I considered it to be a parasitic illness that leeches a person's hope and joy. My objective understanding enabled me to remain nonjudgmental and sincerely offer patients the option to hope when I provided occupational therapy services.

But when I encountered depression face-to-face, my objectivity was lost. The stigma of depression tainted my Spirit and diluted the love Christ extends to all His children, regardless of our psychological condition.

When experiencing severe pain, a person's only goal is relief and hope for recovery. Even those with no religious faith hope healing is possible, especially when they've sought treatment. In the beginning, each time I took Gabapentin and muscle relaxers, I unconsciously hoped I was improving. Though I was unable to resume my activities of daily living, the pain was slightly less intense. I clung to that fraction of relief and longed for a complete recovery. But as time passed, recovery was no longer in sight. I continued taking the medication even though the side effects caused me to teeter on the edges of my life. At the lowest point of my abysmal mental state, depression violated my soul as the fear from the physical pain and my emotional pain took over my thoughts.

When pain and fear combine, they displace hope, erroneously encoding it on each pain pill taken. The brief moments of relief the pills offer create the illusion of hope and recovery. Sadly, hope in a bottle is what many of us who are newly injured cling to. The unrealistic expectation of becoming pain-free and the pills being the only way, intensifies. Desperation accompanies each dose. Then the inseparable connection between severe physical pain and chronic emotional pain muddle rational thoughts.

Studies indicate that chronic pain sufferers have a higher risk of mental health issues, the result of decreased levels of well-being, sleep deprivation, a reduced ability to engage in leisure and employment pursuits, and in personal relationships[42,43]. Regrettably, there is also a 30% to 50% chance of developing depression with the onset of chronic pain and generalized anxiety, even for someone who is not predisposed or has no family history of those types of mental illnesses[44,45].

Knowing my risk of depression, I'd always been watchful of it. But this time, depression snuck up on me. I believed depression's lies—that joy would always be fleeting, recovery was impossible, and pain would control my life.

I knew I felt low, but I couldn't bring myself to acknowledge to anyone that "I" was depressed. It felt like uttering the "D" word was a sin unto itself. That's because for many Christians, admitting to depression is like putting on a scarlet letter of shame. I was blessed and depressed. This statement was no longer an oxymoron. It was my life. I couldn't rally the courage to be vulnerable and admit it out loud. My silence did not make my depression any less real, but it did allow me to hide my detestable reality a little longer.

When family and friends asked how I was doing, I could only bring myself to respond, "I'm getting through it." Towing the line of positivity was my rote response. In the beginning, this was true. But I had to keep up a façade because I was known for being effective in encouraging others and being a woman of faith. I was wedged between shame and pain, unable to free myself from the enemy within.

Depression is a life-threatening thought ideology that doesn't make a sound when it makes invisible emotional cuts that bleed out hope—the spiritual life support and protector against the turbulent notions in our mind.

Spiritually anemic from my emotional wounds, I needed a "spiritual transfusion of hope" to replace the disappointment flowing through my veins. Once depression suppresses the Spirit, our trust in God becomes fragile. Then His divine peace that transcends all understanding becomes inaccessible (Philippians 4:7 NIV).

What I know to be true is that depression is not a weakness, or a stain on an individual's resolve. Depression is the loss of hope—the enduring confidence that joy is attainable in our future. When the anticipation and assured expectation of recovery no longer exists, hope does not exist. Tragically, when hope is gone, the power to move beyond depression to peaceful contentment lies dormant, and depression becomes the silent assassin of the Spirit.

The Merriam-Webster Dictionary defines depression as: "To be lower than the surrounding area, to be pressed down, a hollow place." I was in a hollow place emotionally and spiritually, one where pain, fear, and doubt pressed down on me. My Spirit could not perceive hope. I was spiritually blinded from the darkness within me.

Our spiritual vision is like our natural vision which has a lens that enables us to see objects close and at a distance. Spiritual vision consists of two lenses: a spiritual lens and an eternal lens that enables us to see our circumstances clearly. Unlike human eyes that see objects only as they presently exist, spiritual vision is unbound by time, situation, or illumination. It sees what our human eyes cannot—hope, the substance in faith.

When depression causes these lenses to stop functioning, spiritual blindness occurs. Yet when active, the spiritual lens sees life-altering changes as momentary obstacles within life's lush landscape God has adorned with towering trees, fragrant flowers, breathtaking beaches, and magnificent waterfalls. Through this lens life's unbearable moments are the mountains we climb with God leading the way up and down.

Our spiritual lens operates much like infrared or thermal imaging, which require only heat—not light—to illuminate objects in complete darkness, through fog, snow, and rain. The spiritual lens does its best work in the aforementioned climates. It clearly discerns the warmth from God's faithful love illuminating the path to safe harbor in the darkest storms in our lives.

The eternal lens functions in eternity; it does not function within the constraints of time. Concepts like "early," "late," and "loss" don't exist, because the construct of time rests solely on the foundation of "in time," established by God. His predestined timing is established in Himself for His divine plan to unfold. Life's events occur in seasons and cycles with predetermined beginnings and endings, like winter, spring, summer, fall, and life itself. Therefore, healing and restoration is not early or late. It occurs in God's time.

Our eternal lens perceives time as infinite, understanding that our gains and losses are temporary and occur to position us for what God has planned for us. Through this lens we know that God's blessings are never lost or taken away. His promise of everlasting life, love, grace, comfort, and forgiveness are forever. All the sorrow and pain we encounter on our eternal timeline are resolved by His infinite love.

The grandeur of His predetermined timing is apparent in the masterful orchestration of transitions in the life cycle that begins with conception, streams into birth, progresses through childhood, adolescence, and adulthood, moves into old age, and culminates in everlasting life with our Heavenly Father. At times, He also gifts us with spiritual "aha" moments that allow our spiritual eyes to see His divine strategy when a flashback from our past explains why our lives have unfolded as they have.

Our spiritual vision views our circumstances in life as cycles because not all of life's transitions have unfolded in a typical sequence. Life cycles have many beginnings and endings that culminate on eternity's timeline. We have joyful and sorrowful seasons in our life. Times of abundance and lack. With each ending and beginning we perceive as catastrophic; our spiritual vision views them as turning points which usher us into the next phase in our life. Just as winter yields to spring, our cycles in life should surrender to what comes next without resisting, as exemplified in nature.

When our spiritual and eternal lenses are 20/20, we see like an eagle, recognizing our spiritual and psychological enemies from miles away. As we scan the landscape of pain, we can see depression as a leaf drifting in the wind around our circumstances. We understand that the leaves of depression stem from our emotions of doubt, insecurity, suffering, defeat, and loneliness. With this spiritual discernment we are able to identify the discrepancy in our depressive thoughts and shrewdly see our circumstances for what they are—temporary.

For a while, I could not perceive God's presence while I waited for Him to answer my prayer, to heal me. In the valley of my depression, only the end of my career, the end of my physical abilities, the end of intimacy with my spouse were factual. My reality was a life of constant pain and the end of everything that made me who I thought myself to be.

My vision was blurry. But after much prayer, occasionally my spiritual eyes would refocus as a result of the outpouring of love and support from my family, and I could recognize God was with me. But my spiritual blindness from my depression returned, because the awareness of His loving presence and acceptance of His divine timing had not fully penetrated my entrapped mind and soul.

My spiritual eyesight fully returned on a sunny day as I soaked in lavender-scented bath water. I was reminded of 1 Peter 5:10 NIV that states: ". . . after you have suffered a little while, [God]will himself restore you, and make you strong, firm and steadfast." The word "after" reassured me that God had put my restoration to wholeness on a schedule *He* had planned. My Spirit could see this revelation, and I was able to hope again.

I was fortunate to hear God's call on that icy winter day when I was blind to hope, and my Spirit was on life support. Instead of continuing to hide in my shame, I dragged myself toward the sound of His presence stirring in my soul and moved toward His voice—the same voice that called "Where are you?" in Genesis 3:8-9 NKJV.

When God called me by the name He gave me—"My Beloved Daughter"—He made it impossible for me to ignore Him. The words He spoke during those bathtub encounters broke the chains that bound my Spirit. Hearing His voice when I was spiritually blind saved me. However, that may not always be the case for those blinded by depression or others lost in doubt. They will need help to eliminate the pain that has sealed their spiritual eyelids shut and covered their ears.

After the long delay in my recovery and reaching the depths of my depression I began to seek out God's purpose. The impact of hitting rock bottom shook my entangled thoughts loose. I was better able to see and hear what the Lord was showing me. By His grace, I found my way out of depression's suffocating grip. But this is not always the outcome for those who endure severe pain complicated by emotional anguish. Their future is concealed in their painful present; they see only an onslaught of unknowns that threaten their very existence.

However, in Jesus Christ there is a living hope for a future preserved in eternity. Our current circumstance is not the end of life, just a change in its conditions. Each day presents us with an option to be courageous—to not let depression win. We can choose to hold on to hope that is enduring and steadfast and let go of despair.

To navigate the side effects of chronic pain, it's vital to set realistic expectations that achieving a permanent pain-free life is improbable. Avoid embracing the erroneous ideal that not having the medical condition is the only path to "feel better." There is a middle ground to embrace, a place where recovery is coping, adapting, and accepting physical limitations with the full measure of God's goodness and grace to empower you. This is where one can make peace with a "new normal" and have a fulfilling quality of life.

CHAPTER TWELVE

Doubt

hesitant to believe the truth;
uncertain.

The other "D" word shunned in many Christian circles is doubt. Doubt causes cracks to form in the foundation of faith, which is built on trust in God's Word. Doubt thrives when our trust wavers. Insurmountable fear, pain, loss, spiritual blindness, unanswered questions, and seemingly unanswered prayers makes trusting in God's Word tenuous.

Doubt is an emotional reflex that subverts trust in God while not necessarily undermining a belief in His existence. Yet without trust in Him, we cannot access the lasting peace and comfort available to us by faith. When we doubt our actions are driven by uncertainty and fear. Conversely, with trust in the God's unfailing Word, our actions are driven by faith.

I turned sharply onto the "Doubt Road" when my recovery didn't materialize as expected. Despite praying, my distorted thoughts undermined my full trust in God and caused me to let go of the truth in His word.

But by the grace of God, I uprooted my disbelief by reflecting on His methods and strategies in creating the world and the life within it. My Spirit was reminded that He does nothing without a plan. Every plant, animal, and human being has a purpose, each serving the others in the cycle of life. Humankind and the Earth which sustains our life were planned with precision and intention.

The sudden illness or injury that permanently alters our lives is a surprise only to us. But in the realm of eternity, these life events are a part of a divine plan, one not intended to harm our Spirit or our emotional mind but to transform us into a clearer reflection of His unfailing peace, love, and power. Though we may not agree or fully understand His methods, this type of life cycle is purposed to remind us of our dependence on Him.

I recalled the scripture in Isaiah 55:8–9 NIV, which says: "His thoughts are not our thoughts, and His ways are not our ways and as the heavens are higher than the earth . . . so are His thoughts and His ways higher than ours."

I had to remember my position in this relationship: I am His creation—His child, and He is my God and my Father. Like all children, I didn't always like or agree with my parents' decisions for me, but I had to trust them. It was through them that my well-being was maintained. In the same way it is through God's love, grace, and mercy that our spiritual and emotional well-being is preserved.

As children of God, we believe in His omnipresence and omniscience, but when the sea of life is rough, our emotions overtake us. We abandon our beliefs and forget that He is all-knowing and always with us. We begin to doubt His power and the influence of His presence.

I pondered how Jesus responded to His disciples when they were filled with doubt. He eased their doubt with the authority in His Word and the impact of His Presence.

The synoptic gospels—Mathew, Mark, and Luke—tell the story of Jesus and His disciples traveling to another region by boat. Before they set sail, Jesus told them they were going to the other side of the lake. A storm developed and worsened while Jesus slept. Naturally, the disciples became afraid as the waves and winds violently tossed the boat. In Mathew 8:23–27 NIV the disciples shout, "Lord, save us!" In Mark 4:38–41 NIV they wake Jesus, accusing Him of not caring if they drowned. And in Luke 8:24–25 NIV they told Jesus they were drowning. Jesus spoke to the wind and waves, calming them. Then He asked the disciples what happened to their faith and why were they afraid.

I believe God asks the same questions of us today: Why don't we trust Him when we are fearful and anxious? How has the veracity of His Word and His professed and proven love for us become unreliable to us?

The disciples panicked. Consumed by the force of the tumultuous waves, pelting rain, roaring thunder, flashing lightening, and howling winds, they could focus only on what their natural eyes could see and what their physical bodies felt. They feared for their lives. Their emotions overcame them. They forgot—or didn't trust—the plan Jesus gave them when they were on solid ground.

Their confrontation with the possibility of death ushered in disbelief and weakened their confidence in Jesus—the living hope in front of them. The peaceful sleeping Jesus did not reassure them that all was well.

Their fear caused them to revert to how they'd coped with storms before Jusus entered their lives: They relied on their own knowledge and survival skills as fishermen to navigate the storm. But when they reached the limits of their expertise they called to Jesus for help and accused Him of not caring.

We are no different from the disciples. When faced with unsettling circumstances and our well-being is in jeopardy, we are equally as forgetful and blinded by fear. Doubt prevails, we don't account for the presence of God, and if we are frightened enough we may even accuse Him, too. At times we also default to our hardwired patterns for self-preservation by relying on our intellect, resources, and influence to fix the situation. But when our ability fails to resolve the problem and our egos are humbled, then we seek His presence.

When the storm was raging, I also noticed the disciples believed Jesus was unaware and unconcerned about their grave situation because he did not respond to storm with the same fear as they had. He was resting peacefully while they were anxious and afraid.

Again, we are just like the disciples. We tend to attribute God's silence or delayed response to a lack of concern for us. Not only is this not true, but it is a direct contradiction of God's motives. He cares deeply for us; we are His creation, designed to be in a glorious relationship with Him. He created humanity in His image and sent Jesus to be the outstretched bridge we cross to inherit eternal life with Him.

God's silence and delayed response are purposed to bring us closer to Him so we can listen more carefully to what He has said and be comforted by His presence while we wait for what He will say. God calls us to be nearer to Him so we can take hold of the peace, strength, and wisdom He desires to impart to us during the storms in life.

When we are in a storm He has not chosen to end, the storm is where God wants us to be. He wants us to see with our spiritual eyes and know that a treacherous storm is only a threat to capsize our lives. He wants us to trust that the threat of harm cannot keep us from the promise in the Word he gave concerning us. Romans 11:29 AMP* tells us He does not change His mind about His plans for us. God wants our response to the storms in life to show our trust in Him. He wants to see if panic and doubt will abound—or the power in His word abound.

Hopefully, we will remember that a storm in life is not a life-threatening storm with Jesus Christ on board. His presence changes everything. When we acknowledge His presence with us, the storm loses its foreboding power, becoming docile wind and moisture in the air. When we encounter life's storms and difficult terrains, we must remember to model Jesus's trust in God through his surrendered prayer when He was in Gethsemane. He said, "not my will but yours be done" (Luke 22:42 NIV).

A time may come when the sharp edges of life fray the tightly woven fibers of our faith. Though our physical and emotional pain may momentarily cause our faith to falter and land us in the den of depression and doubt, our duty is to recognize that God does not intend for us to stay in the environment that makes it difficult for us to trust Him. He desires us to fervently seek His truth and perceive His presence.

When I asked God to reveal Himself to me more fully and to guide me, I surrendered my expectations about what His resolution would be. I had to trust in His integrity and wait for insight and revelation. I positioned myself to be at peace with the possibility that physical relief might always be fleeting, yet His grace would be sufficient and sustain me. To reclaim my faith, I held onto my hope in Christ with both hands and stopped listening to the doubt that infiltrated my emotions.

To overcome doubt, I embraced the unseen evidence of my faith, which is anchored in the reliabilty of God's promises. I recognized that doubt distorts God's promise by dulling our spiritual awareness of the

---

* . . . the gifts and the calling of God are irrevocable (for He does not withdraw what He has given nor does He change His mind about those to whom He gives His grace or to whom He sends His call)

Heavenly place He has given us (Ephesians 2:6 AMP)[†]. Often, doubt fills the elevated seat our trust in God once occupied. When doubt reigns, uncertainty erodes the foundation of faith.

Our Doubt Says:

God, I hear what you have said but it does not match my circumstances.
I have been through a lot. My pain and my anxiety are real. I can't see, feel, or find the everlasting peace and confidence You have spoken of.
God, I do not know if You can bridge this gap between us.
This gap between Your comfort and my anguish.
Help me find You.
Help me see You.
Help me experience Your grace that You said that I've had since the day I accepted Christ, my Lord, My God.
Help me with the unbelief that is smothering my faith.
I have believed You before and I want to believe You again, but it is hard.
I have seen what You have done in some of our past experiences.
I have seen what You have done in other people's lives
But I am having a difficult time gathering the crumbs of my faith—because my circumstances have tied my hands behind my back.
Free me!

But God Says:

I know the plans I have for you.
Plans to prosper you and not harm you
Plans to give you hope and a future (Jeremiah 29:11 NIV)

---

† . . . seated us with Him in the heavenly places . . .

Doubt

Do you believe Me?

Do not give up your seat of hope. It is still in the Heavenly Place I prepared for you.

I know the twists, turns, and physical pain you are experiencing has caused you to trip and fall, but if you

Reach for Me

I will stretch out My hand to you.

I will stand you up.

Come to Me with all your burdens and I will give you rest (Mathew 11:28 NIV).

Stay with Me and you will see that I have honored My promise to you.

Let go of your doubt. Hold on to My true word instead.

Trust Me more than you trust your fear.

Let the rising sun and your beating heart confirm that I AM with you.

God's merciful response to our doubt is to reveal Himself fully through His perfect record of faithfulness. If we believe in Him more than we believe our doubt, then we regain our seat beside Him and our enemy within becomes our footstool. I discarded my doubt and picked up His word to dispel the falsehood in my fears. He lovingly wrapped His mercy around me and dispelled my doubt with His truth. I remembered and believe all that God says we are:

God's workmanship (Ephesians 2:10 KJV)[‡]
His Chosen (Ephesians 1:4-5 NIV)[§]
A Citizen of Heaven (Philippians 3:20)[¶]

[‡] For we are Gods' workmanship . . .

[§] For he chose us in him before the creation of the world to be holy and blameless in his sight . . . through Jesus Christ

[¶] . . . our citizenship is in heaven . . .

Do not allow doubt to steal God's promises. Stretch your arms farther and seek His presence and His truth with all your might. Leave your grief, disappointment, and despair with Him, the Prince of Peace, and He will comfort you (Isaiah 9:6 NIV)**. Do not hold onto those emotions because they corrupt you, the vessel carrying it.

The wounds incurred from pierced faith hemorrhage both hope and trust, and only the ultimate Healer can restore them. Only Christ can remedy injured hope masquerading as depression and injured faith camouflaged as doubt. Seek God's Word by praying from the Spirit within you that intimately knows Him. I plead with you to call on His presence to engulf your senses, flooding every crevasse of your mind, body, and Spirit with guaranteed wholeness. Do not allow debilitating physical, mental, and spiritual pain separate you from the gift, the inheritance of everlasting life and love that He has given to all His children (Romans 8:38–39)††.

According to Luke 22:32 NIV, Jesus prays our faith will not fail. He is seated on the right hand of our Heavenly Father interceding for us. He is advocating for us and praying we overcome our trials and tribulations. He is praying that we hold on to the hope that He secured for us. He is praying that we always trust in His love and eternal plans for us. Trust God enough to get you over to the other side of your injury, diagnosis, or disease. He is greater than your pain. Greater than your fear. Greater than your anxiety. Greater than your disappointment. Keep the words

---

** . . . And he will be called Wonderful Counselor, Mighty God, Everlasting Father, Prince of Peace

†† . . . Neither death nor life . . . neither present not the future . . . neither height nor depth, nor anything else in all creation will be able to separate us from the love of God that is in Christ Jesus our Lord.

of 1 Peter 5:7 NIV readily available to remind your anxious soul to—
"Cast all your anxiety upon Him because he cares for you."

Live courageously with these truths and keep the spiritual and emotional mind focused on Him to access peace, hope, strength, and protection from the collateral effects of chronic pain (Isaiah 26:3-4 AMP)‡‡.

---

‡‡ . . . Keep in perfect and constant peace the one whose minds are steadfast [committed and focused on You ..] because he trusts in You

CHAPTER THIRTEEN

Support System

*The people who provide practical
and emotional support*

If you know someone with a sudden debilitating injury or pain-inducing disease who has been prescribed opiate or antiepileptic medications like Gabapentin and Lyrica, know they are undergoing a significant change in their life. Spend time with them; your presence could be the visual life raft they are looking up to as they are drifting in the abyss of uncertainty and depression.

Having a "support system" can be a lifesaver for someone caught in chronic pain's web. When my recovery stalled the rollercoaster of emotions disoriented my orientation of whom God called me to be in this situation and who He was. The unraveling of my faith began when I collided with the wall of unmet expectations. This collision caused my hope to fail and the secure place in my soul where my trust in God once occupied collapsed. This void in my soul created an opening for depression to creep in.

This could be the same juncture for the undoing of your loved one as well. They will need your help. Your relationship with your loved one positions you to become their support system. Have the courage to reach out to them and let them know how important they are to you.

Despite the huge benefits of seeing a mental health provider, it's often difficult to access professional care. It is for this reason the role of a support network, be it a group or a singular friend, is invaluable.

As the support system, you should approach your loved one from a place of compassion and concern, one in which you suspend expectations, opinions, and judgment about their emotional and spiritual response to their personal crisis. Give them an opportunity to express their thoughts and feelings. They need the space to be angry, sad, and disappointed so they can begin the work of confronting the emotional enemies within.

It is imperative that you are sensitive to your loved one's emotional state. Remember that their life has imploded, and you are like a guidepost, pointing them toward the exit from the twisted and treacherous road of pain and depression. Whether your loved one is or isn't willing to talk to you, encourage them to see a therapist to get professional coping strategies.

~

As an occupational therapist I routinely develop strategic plans and tools to help clients and their support systems achieve positive outcomes. I created the *I Am Here for You Pact*© to equip individuals and their support persons with strategies to address the emotional challenges inherent in disabling chronic pain. This tool establishes a framework for the support person and their loved one to communicate.

It is designed to foster a resolution for "low frequency" emotions like fear, despair, and loneliness, by using journaling and charting as a means for reflection, introspection, discussion, and establishing a solution. The

Pact includes many faith-based principles, but these elements can be omitted if they don't align with your loved one's beliefs.

Because your loved one is emotionally vulnerable, the *Pact* requires the support person to have integrity, self-control, and neutrality. Should you react with anger, frustration, or a demeaning attitude, your loved one will no longer trust you with their inner most thoughts. They will shut down and suffer alone in silence.

The *I Am Here for You Pact*© is a proactive intervention for a support network. It should be established at the onset of an injury or diagnosis, to provide a foundation for open communication about depression and discouragement. If the *Pact* cannot be initiated at the start, implement the *Pact* as soon as possible.

To begin, the support person reminds the loved one how much they mean to them and those around them. Then they introduce the *Pact* by explaining its purpose and criteria: to foster mutual understanding and commitment.

The *Pact* Agreement Fundamentals:

1. Do some research about the condition your loved one is experiencing.

2. The support person agrees to never judge, blame, or shame the loved one. They agree to adhere to the judgment-free zone to maintain the *Pact* integrity.

3. The loved one agrees to be honest and communicate if a change occurs in their positive and/or hopeful outlook.

4. The loved one agrees to refrain from what I call the emotional shutdown avoidance tactic, and to have difficult conversations to communicate their overwhelming feelings and frightening thoughts.

5. The loved one agrees to develop a plan to address those thoughts and emotions.

6. When the *Pact* transitions from a theoretical plan to an active intervention to dismantle grief, loss, and depression, the loved one agrees to consider reaching for hope instead of defeat.

7. The loved one and the support person agree to hold themselves accountable to the *Pact*.

Below is the structure to establish the *I Am Here for You Pact* Agreement©

The Support Person/*Pact* Friend

1. The support person should introduce the Pact from a place of compassion by saying, "I know you are experiencing the physical and emotional impact of your condition and that you are fighting this situation alone. But I love you and want to join you in the fight. I want to be there for you if or when things become difficult."

2. The role of the support person is to listen and allow your loved one to cry as long and loudly as they need to. As much as you may wish to, you cannot rush them into feeling better. Their recovery is on God's timeline, not yours or theirs.

3. Listen more than you speak. Don't become uncomfortable with the awkward silent pauses in the conversation. Instead, acknowledge the silence, so your loved one doesn't feel pressured to speak or to comfort you. You can say, "It is okay that you don't have much to say right now. Often, I don't know what to

say either. I'm just thankful we can be together and that I can support you in this moment."

4. Actively listen and acknowledge the physical/emotional losses they share and the emotional toll it's having on them. You might say, "I cannot imagine how you're feeling. But I believe you when you say _____" (This is when you repeat the thoughts/feelings they shared with you.) This is the use of "reflection," an excellent therapeutic technique, to show you understand what is being said without judgment.

5. Set an appointed time to be physically present with them often. Or have a scheduled video call with them if you cannot meet in person.

6. Show you can be trusted with their emotions by:
   a. Being patient. If they become anxious or irritated during a conversation and don't explain their feelings well. Do not pressure them to be "more specific." It can be difficult to articulate complex emotional thoughts. Instead, accept that you may not understand how they feel and listen.
   b. Do your best to avoid interrupting when they are speaking.
   c. Don't use anything they share to demean them.

7. Don't condemn them; God is not judging them. He is patiently waiting for them to recognize His presence. You should patiently wait too.

8. Be aware of the Stages of Grief: Denial, Anger, Bargaining, Depression and Acceptance. Research the stages online. Share what you learn with them. This information could provide much needed emotional insight.

9. Be patient. Give them time to work through the stages of grief. There is no specific order or timeframe for the stages. The one exception is that acceptance is the last stage. Don't try to rush the process.

10. Don't hypothesize about God's intention for your loved one. That revelation can occur only between them and God. Remind them that you are like Aaron and Hur, who held up Moses's arms when he became tired so they would be victorious on the battlefield (Exodus 17:11-15 NIV). You are holding up your loved one when they become fatigued during the battle for their quality of life. You are their support to help them triumph.

11. Don't try to fix them. Your suggestions are just that, suggestions. Don't feel offended if your loved one doesn't implement your suggestions. As much as you want to "fix" them, you cannot. The timeframe for their grief and healing is an internal process. You are there to provide external love, encouragement, and support—to help lift them up when they are sinking. Stay constant, even if it seems like your efforts are not helping. Do not become discouraged. A faithful friend or family member can make the difference between permanent and temporary emotional paralysis. You are the friend helping them get in the room with Jesus (Mark 2:1-12 NIV)*.

12. Avoid telling them how to feel or respond. "Should" statements convey judgment and correction and cause others to feel guilty and withdraw from you, regardless of your good intentions.

---

* . . . some men came, bringing a paralyzed man . . . Since they could not get him to Jesus because of the crowd, they made an opening in the roof above Jesus by digging through it and then lowered . . . the mat the man was lying on. When Jesus saw their faith, he said to the paralyzed man ". . . your sins are forgiven. . . . get up, take your mat and go home . . ." He got up . . . and walked out . . .

13. Empathy is better than sympathy. Sympathy expresses sadness for your loved one. But it's often based on what you imagine in your thoughts about what they're feeling. Sympathy says: "I know you must be hurting, and I feel sorry for you." But empathy engages your heart. You put yourself in their shoes. You sit in the seat of loss they are sitting in and emotionally connect with their pain. Empathy says: "I know you must be hurting, and I cannot feel what you're experiencing. But I'd feel angry and disappointed if I were hurting all the time and I'd be distressed if I couldn't do simple things for myself too."

14. Now that you are more knowledgeable about lingering loss and grief from an acute condition that becomes permanent, you can ask open-ended questions. You could start by saying, "Injuries and or medical conditions like yours can make it hard to adjust." Avoid asking, "How are you doing?" because that question allows someone to hide the loss and doubt they're experiencing. Instead, ask questions like the ones below to begin in-depth conversations to better support them and understand their feelings.

    a. "How are you dealing with the sudden change in your life that has not allowed you to resume your normal activities? Go to the places you went before? Not allowed you to work? To sleep? Or do the things you enjoy?"

    b. Use reflection and say "I know you miss being able to _____" (repeat what they have shared they miss doing). Then say, "I can only glimpse the pain that you allow me to see, and I cannot fathom how your loss must weigh on you. But I love you too much to leave you alone. I want to help you get through this." "How can I support you?" "How can I help you?"

    c. "Have you stopped trusting God?"

15. The power of prayer is unmatched. Activate that power by praying with your loved one or privately on their behalf. Pray that their Spirit will be positioned to receive the revelation God has prepared for them. Only He knows His purpose for our trials. Pray for them to have the strength and endurance to withstand the time it takes for their deliverance. Pray that the foundation of their faith will be reinforced by the truth of God's Word.

The Loved One

1. Begin to journal daily—or at least weekly—during your recovery. This is a wonderful outlet to acknowledge and express the range of emotions you're experiencing. Writing down your thoughts provides a wider vantage point to better process them. When your emotions are on paper, they are in full view for you to not just feel them, but to see them. When you can see the emotional enemies within it is easier to confront them and free yourself from them. When you can see the enemies within it easier to fight them.

2. Create the *Emotion Chart*. It's designed to help you address the daunting emotions that interfere with your mental well-being. It's the action plan in the *Pact* to help you create specific strategies to expose and overcome overwhelming thoughts and feelings. Because it's difficult to talk about emotions you're not proud of, the chart also provides a written tool your support person can read to better understand your feelings. Together, you can then develop strategies to diffuse those thoughts should they surface again.

3. To set up the chart, turn a sheet of paper horizontally. The chart will have three columns and five rows spaced to cover the entire sheet. Make three equally spaced columns by drawing two vertical lines from the top edge of the page to the bottom edge of the page. Make five equally spaced rows by drawing four horizontal lines from the left edge of the paper to the right edge. Draw an additional narrower row at the top for the headings. In the heading space, label the left column "Emotions," the middle column "Date," and the right column "Strategy." In the Emotion column, list your "low-frequency" emotions or thoughts such as—anger, doubt, worthlessness, hopelessness. In the "Date" column, list the date you have decided to confront the listed emotions. This is the date you have chosen to expose your inner thoughts to immutable truths. This is the date you reclaim your power. Write the date on the corresponding row for each emotion. This may also be the same date you choose to share the chart with your *Pact Friend*. In the Strategy column, list the strategy or solution to address and diffuse each corresponding emotion.

When someone's coping strategy involves hiding their true feelings, it allows fear, anxiety, and depression to continually recycle—tormenting your loved one. Without a resource such as the *I Am Here for You Pact*©, which fosters communication with a support network and emotional self-awareness, internal healing is obstructed.

As you step into the role of a *Support Person/Pact Friend*, keep in mind the scripture in Jude 1:22: "Be merciful to those who doubt." Embrace compassion for those who struggle with doubt, depression,

OUD, SUD, and other mental illness. Recognize the courage it takes to share fears, grief, and failure with a professional—let alone someone you love. So discard judgment when your loved one shares their despair.

CHAPTER FOURTEEN

Faith

trust you can rely on; complete trust;
secure trust; trustworthy

I can understand how, for those who don't embrace the tenets of Christian faith, the notion of relying on the promises of God instead of on medical experts is like making a wish. But my personal encounter with God transformed my faith and perspective on healing.

I realized that placing my hope for healing in prescriptions was a form of wishful thinking. Limited relief that expired every four to six hours proved this avenue for recovery was unsustainable. I was dying from a "psychological cardiac arrest" brought on by depression and physical pain. I needed a deep, inner revival to reach the divide between my mind and Spirit. This "internal resuscitation" could only be accessed through faith.

Although I'd always relied on faith during difficult times, practicing faith while enduring aggressive confrontational pain was entirely different. Pain affected every facet of my existence—from the physical aspects of living to my psychological framework for coping. It shook the foundation of faith that was incubated in my youth.

My belief in God was the extent of my faith. Although belief is essential to faith, it is only the formative stage. Only complete trust in God produces mature, sustaining faith. This experience exposed my immature belief system and taught me how to securely rely on God.

I asked myself: Why had I survived this life-changing event that could have resulted in a slow death from a substance use disorder or a chronic incapacitating depression? Given that chronic back pain is the leading contributor to disability in 160 countries, a bulging disc is hardly unique[46]. With reflection, I was able to gain a broader perspective than that of pain's impact on me and my family. I realized my experience held spiritual and societal insights that could benefit others.

Although I'm not a theologian, I was able to clearly see the spiritual and emotional traps which arise from severe long-term pain that was initially expected to be temporary. When a productive life collides with a chronic pain diagnosis it causes a physical, emotional, and spiritual tsunami that has life-threatening consequences.

Severe pain can destabilize belief and cause us to misunderstand God's Word and His character. When the plans and expectations our ego constructed fail, we become empty vessels. This void will be filled with either hope or despair.

I thought about Jesus's grief prior to his surrender, captivity, and crucifixion. Reflecting on our Savior's torturous pain and suffering triggered condemnation in my Spirit, because in no way was I suffering like that. I asked myself what I was really grieving. The pain, obviously, but the loss of whom I'd thought myself to be was tormenting me. My fabricated identity was dying and trying to survive.

Prior to my injury, my ego and complacent faith were on autopilot. But I could not be whom God wanted me to be with this form of faith. My ego had to die so my Spirit could live fully with the trust in God as my foundation.

My faith grew alongside my ego, much like weeds growing in a garden alongside flowers. My ego had become intertwined with my faith, and I was unknowingly overrun with weeds of arrogance. Thankfully, the Master Gardener intervened and tilled the soil of my life. He uprooted the weeds and discarded the immature fruit produced from my self-confidence and intellect. The mature fruit of faith God intended for me to produce in the next stage of my life would be grown by His diligent, faithful hand.

Although my faith was lacking, I was able to access God's eternal reserve of spiritual resources that He provides for all His children. Spending time in God's presence and recommitting to His Word offset the damage the bulging disc and depression had on my soul.

Pain uncovers an unpopular truth that our immature faith fails to acknowledge: God's will does not always feel good. To fulfill God's purpose, we will be uncomfortable in several seasons of our life. To be a child of God is to carry Christ's banner and represent Him in all we do and how we respond to burdensome circumstances. Because of the grace He has bestowed upon us, we have the stamina to withstand the weight of heartache, pain, and disability. We must remember when difficult times arise, they will not permanently diminish the joy He has sealed in us.

Just as we want our children to display strong family principals, God wants us to do the same: to understand that our burdens can be lightened with Him by our side. This is shown through our faith, which is apparent in our perspective, attitude, and actions during troubling seasons. He wants His goodness to be evident to those we encounter.

The scripture, "Faith is the substance of things hoped for, the evidence of things not seen" (Hebrews11:1 NKJV), forms the pillar of faith. But our error is basing our hopes on what we want God to do for us, and not on God's promises to us.

A problem for many of us is anchoring hope on our expectations of how and when we think God should answer our prayers, rather than on His timing for the revelation of His Word in our situation. As a result we do not see the evidence of faith because it is entangled with our expectations of what we believe we deserve and when we should receive it.

This perspective blinds us to the blessings God has given us while we wait for His response to our pleas. When the wait is long, we begin to judge God as untrustworthy or unloving and blame ourselves for not being "good enough" for God to fulfill our heartfelt requests. Sadly, in both instances, we are wrong.

Emotional and physical pain makes it difficult for us to understand that a delayed answer from God means He has given us the answer, but we don't recognize it. Or, He is teaching us to trust Him longer for our faith to mature so we can perceive His answer. Trusting God over an extended period, even when it seems impossible for our psychological and physical pain to end, is the true manifestation of the faith He desires us to attain. The need for pain to end expediently erodes the power in faith that comes from patiently waiting.

Chronic pain does not end. It increases and decreases as the nervous system automates or may lie dormant until a physical or emotional event triggers it. This doesn't mean God hasn't answered our prayers for deliverance. It means He is waiting for us to recognize what He has told us about enduring and to reach for the promise of peace He has already given us.

If we can be aware of our tendency to filter our hope and faith through our own desires and timeframe, we can avoid the disappointment of what we deem to be an unanswered prayer. We can position ourselves to better understand that the purpose of tribulation is to increase our faith and deepen our relationship with God.

Severe chronic pain and its sidekick, depression, have a way of separating our hope and faith—two elements that cannot function unless bonded together. They are as inseparable as blood flow is to oxygen, which sustains our life. Oxygen is carried in our blood, keeping all the systems in our body functioning. Without the oxygen in our blood, it is impossible for us to remain alive. In the same way, without hope—the oxygen in our faith—it is impossible for our Spirit to remain alive in the condition God intended.

Knowing that hope is the indispensable substance in faith that sustains our spiritual and emotional well-being, we should be more prudent about where we place our hope.

After I retrieved my hope from the medications and placed it in God restoring me, the intensity of my emotional pain lessened. I aligned myself with God's expectations of me to access the eternal healing He provides. I meditated daily on Romans 12:12 NIV, which says: "Be joyful in hope, patient in affliction, faithful in prayer." When I prayed, I heard God saying:

"Daughter, I will heal you, but your physical pain will linger so you can come to know the power of My peace when you completely trust me. As I heal your mind, you will begin to feel better."

Partially trusting God does not give us full access to His peace or His grace. To believe in God is to trust God. This trust makes it possible for us to access the His abundant and sufficient grace, which sustains us in difficult times. When we trust that God is keeping His promise to never abandon His children and that He will always provide, allows us to accept God's answer for chronic pain to remain. We know He is providing a refuge for us amid physical suffering—a refuge found in His peace and promise that our physical suffering is temporary in our eternal timeline.

But when we doubt God's promise to provide peace that surpasses our present conditions and circumstances, we abandon His promise of peace when we need it most. In doing so, we may believe that the presence of pain and hard times equals the absence of His love. But when our faith is built on a foundation of truth, we will accept as fact Matthew 28:20 NIV, which says: ". . . And surely I am with you always, to the very end of the age." We will acquiesce to the purpose and intention of difficult times knowing that pain and disappointment do not impact God's divine plan for us.

To align with His purpose, I had to ask God: What do You want me to do? To learn? To see? How does my current circumstance benefit Your Kingdom's purpose for my life? How do You want me to be transformed?

I began to reflect on scriptures about patience and suffering, such as James 1:2–4 NIV[*] and Romans 5:3–4 AMP[†]. Those scriptures reminded me that I should remain hopeful during this time of tribulation because a trial of faith produces patience, perseverance, and character. Had my chronic pain ended, patience and perseverance would not been able to complete their perfect work in me. His plan for my faith to mature and for me to develop a closer relationship with Him more fully would have been interrupted, and my spiritual growth delayed.

---

[*] Consider it pure joy . . . whenever you face trials . . . because you know that the testing of your faith produces perseverance. Let perseverance finish its work so that you may be mature and complete, not lacking anything.

[†] . . . but [with joy] let us exalt in our sufferings and rejoice in our hardships, knowing that hardship (distress, pressure, trouble) produces patient endurance; and endurance proven character . . . hope and confident assurance [of eternal salvation].

The expectation felt by many with chronic pain is wanting God to remove the physical pain. However, I had to recognize that since God had not entirely eliminated my physical pain, this chronic pain situation is where He wanted me to be so I could experience the power of His peace and receive the provision of His wholeness that resulted in relief from my emotional pain.

I had to discard my fixed notions that restoration would look like a full return of my former abilities. Waiting for God, I realized He is not in the business of restoring what was; He is in the business of making us a new creation, one that accurately reflects His character and image.

Immersed in the comfort of His presence, I got closer to restoration. I needed His presence more than my perfect recovery plan. I knew I had to wait for the new seeds of my hope to germinate and develop an underground network of densely rooted faith.

I'd been confident that my faith prior to my injury was reliable. It was always readily accessible and had ushered me through my difficult times. But my reaction to the bulging disc didn't follow my playbook for overcoming disappointment, loss, rejection, and sadness. This injury was a trial by fire. God the healer, God the provider, God the omnipotent, God the omniscient, and God the omnipresent got lost in my emotions and feelings.

But God loves us so much that he has given us weapons to protect our Spirit and our mind—spiritual weapons readily accessible to defend our souls. He gave us the belt of truth, the breastplate of righteousness, the shield of faith, the helmet of salvation, and the sword with the Word from the Spirit. I'd gotten comfortable claiming I would never take my armor off, but I did. I was temporarily unprotected in this spiritual battle.

Because of God's divine provision, the attack from my circumstances triggered my spiritual armor that was forged by the Holy Spirit to activate.

I learned that experiencing tribulation is necessary for refined faith to develop. This battle increased my faith and renewed my fellowship with God. I reflected again on Luke 22:32 when Jesus spoke to Peter about his failed faith. The Amplified version says, "but I have prayed for you . . . , that your faith [and confidence in Me] may not fail; and once you have turned back again [to Me], strengthen and support your brothers [in the faith]." I am eternally grateful that Jesus prayed for me as well. I am grateful that I trusted Him and turned back to Him again.

~

My experience revealed aspects of the Christian perspective I had not considered before. We attest to God's omnipotence and omniscience but demand when, where, and how we should be restored. In doing this, we allow disbelief and resentment to supersede our trust in God when the outcomes of our circumstances don't align with our expectations.

We judge God for not preventing or ending agonizing conditions in a timeframe we've deemed reasonable. When we are in distress we quickly forget our position in the relationship. We are the creation of the Creator, children of the Almighty God. We have been set apart and chosen to complete the good works prepared in advance (Eph 2:10 NIV)‡. The judgment we place on God contradicts our acknowledgement of God's sovereign and infinite latitude to orchestrate our lives in accordance with His purpose.

Our inability to accept and understand that His ways are not our ways and His thoughts are not our thoughts, creates a gap in our faith that our wavering emotions fill (Isaiah 55:8-9 NIV). Our uncertainty

‡ For we are God's handiwork, created in Christ Jesus to do good works, which God prepared in advance for us to do.

and doubt lead the charge of defamation against the Creator. Our distorted ideals such as: God should protect us from loss; God should not allow tragedy; and God should change our diagnosis reinforce a faulty belief system that undermines our ability to respond with assured faith.

Our flawed beliefs ignore the excruciating process that fulfilled God's love for us through Jesus Christ suffering and how that process applies to us, the children of God. Meaning, we will also have to endure for God's Word, God's purpose to be fulfilled in us (Isaiah 55:11 NIV).

The torture Christ suffered illustrates that pain is a part of life—but not the end of life. Christ's torment on the cross was purposed for our salvation. Our pain also has a purpose. My injury was a necessary means to transform my faith. Through this process, I came to understand that pain and disability are a temporary state of being we pass through as we travel toward everlasting life.

I believe that if we reflect on Jesus's emotions and prayers at Gethsemane prior to his crucifixion and model his response, we will receive an overflow of peace and power as we surrender to the deliverance God has purposed in our chronic pain condition.

Jesus was deeply distressed by what was going to unfold. He prayed three times for God to change the path before him. Even though his prayers were sorrowful, God did not give Jesus what he asked for. Jesus knew the crucifixion was the plan God intended. He knew the brutal and torturous process was the only means for God's plan to be fulfilled (Isaiah 53:5; 1 Peter 2:24, 3:18; Rev 13:8 NIV). His fear did not compromise His trust in God to deliver Him when the process was over. Jesus surrendered to God's will. We are called to do the same, to obey His word, to always trust only in Him, and surrender to His will for us.

As a part of the body of Christ we are not exempt from enduring unfathomable situations. I believe God would not call us conquerors if there were nothing we had to conquer. Our command as His Chosen and Dearly Loved is to endure in faith and persevere in hope regardless of the extenuating conditions in our physical body and the external circumstances in our life.

But when we grow in our discontent with the circumstances God has permitted, our diminished hope and faith lead to toxic disappointment covering our exposed egos and broken hearts. This disappointment becomes fertile ground for chronic pain and depression to uproot faith when God has not done what we prayed for. These conditions cultivate doubt, which proliferates in the dense forest in the mind, concealing the Tree of Life God planted within us.

If the eyes of our heart could perceive that God's presence and Jesus Christ's sacrifice are the expressions of God's love for us, we would know that it is always through hardship that we learn His grace is sufficient. When our trust prompts us to rely on Him more completely, we can take hold of the full measure of His grace, and it becomes easier to accept deliverance on His terms—not ours.

We forget that as followers of Christ our lives are purposed for His glory. Humbly we give Him credit when things go well. But we forget that when they don't, we should still reflect His faithfulness and goodness. When life feels bad, and death, loss, and immeasurable pain arise, we must be alert to examine our thoughts and emotions to ensure they align with His faithful love toward us. When our thoughts and emotions do not agree with the truth in His word, we should quickly discard them.

As I looked in the mirror of my disbelief, I saw the reflection of my Godlike tendencies staring back at me. And what a shameful sight it was. Being created in His image as an autonomous human being, we think we have total control over the outcomes in our life. We believe recovery, healing, our careers, and life plans are carried out on our terms; we decide what we will and won't do. To a point, this is true and our

Godlike ego is affirmed. The effort we put into something equates with the results we receive, but not always.

In our faith-based relationship, God's will and God's plan are the defining variables in the outcomes in our life, and it's often the one we distort. Under the shroud of emotion and pain, it's easy to forget that our circumstances have been set by God. He allows and restricts. He alone sets the terms that our egos attempt to manipulate. When our efforts fail, we blame God, ourselves, those closest to us, or anyone who may have a role in the problem. We forget to seek God first to gain insight and revelation about the situation. With our emotions and egos leading us, we distort God's intent.

Then our God-like posture allows us to assume our relationship with God is on-demand, transactional. We pray, make requests, and expect Him to deliver. We frequently forget our agreement with God when we accepted Christ' sacrifice, becoming His chosen ones. God is the CEO and Jesus Christ is the brand we represent. We don't get to bend the terms and conditions of our relationship. He alone determines when, how, and where life's "storms" arise to perfect our faith. God's timing is never based on our ideas of who, what, or when our circumstances change. They are always based on His divine plan.

In our relationship with God, our transactional beliefs are further perpetuated in our conditional hope. When we don't receive the "thing" we asked for our hope fades. We misuse hope as means to expect to receive what we "need" from God—needs that are often in the form of objects and not His presence. However, the power in hope is available only through our trust in the presence of God. Hope in God is the anchor keeping us from flailing to-and-fro when physical and emotional pain suddenly overwhelm us. It is our hope—our trust—that enables us to wait on God's timing for the resolution in life's dilemmas.

I believe that spiritual and emotional wholeness is one of God's many remarkable blessings. With the gift of the Holy Spirit, we have access to immeasurable peace and joy untouched by our physical circumstances. God wants our faith and mental well-being to be invulnerable to the downsides of life, including terminal diagnoses, chronic pain, and disability

We will all have times when we experience our own Garden of Gethsemane—a place where our faith and obedience are pressed. God wants us to accept that He is greater than our circumstances. To accept that His "No" to our prayers is because a "Yes" doesn't align with His divine plan. He wants us to know that we can be in a painful situation yet have peace, and that despair and misery are not a product of His fruit—they are the fruit of fear and doubt. He wants us to always know and hold on to the fruit of His Spirit—hope, peace, faithfulness, patience, and joy.

He wants us to accept that our anger, fear, disappointment, and despair are not intended to reside within us permanently. Those emotions are a reflex in distressing circumstances. They should be short-lived and not change our perspective on His love and plan for our eternal lives.

We should model how Jesus handled his emotions in the the Garden of Gethsemane. In prayer, He tearfully expressed His distressing emotions to God and did not allow His fear to deter Him from following God's plan.

We must remember: God grows our faith in the troubled waters in life. As He reveals Himself more fully, He intends our faith to develop deep roots from our trust in Him—not in the props from a good life. He desires for us to have faith that can withstand turbulent seasons of pain and loss. A faith that provides abundant, unassailable peace that is impenetrable from life's sorrows.

When I relinquished my expectation and reached for His extended hand, I tore down my shrine built on optimism, expectations, expertise, and conditional hope. When I stopped taking the medication and stripped away doubt and fear, I accessed the wholeness God offered. The consistency and reliability of the Word of God that has been unvarnished by time was the path I chose to follow. Once peace prevailed despite the presence of chronic physical pain, I attained faith that was unswayed by my circumstance, and I said this prayer to my Redeemer to remain immersed in the wholeness and contentment He intended:

"Heavenly Father, remind my Spirit of Your priorities when I place my priorities above Yours—when my life gets busy and when my emotions get the best of me. Remind my Spirit of Your priorities when my circumstances hide Your promise for my life . . . Your promise to never leave me . . . and that You chose me, called me Yours, and redeemed me. Remind me of Your grace when my situation hides Your authority in this world and my life. Remind me, God, to keep my eyes and my thoughts on You and not be shaken by the disturbing changes happening around me. Not be disturbed the the changes in my health. Remind me that You use life and death, joy and despair, and times of peace and chaos for Your divine purpose. Remind me of the miraculous birth, life, death, and resurrection of Jesus Christ, my Lord and Savior.

"Fill my heart, my mind, and my Spirit with joy and peace. I thank You and I praise You, God, for loving me so. Give me the wisdom, courage, and humility to acquiesce to Your plans, Your purpose, and Your will and to lay my plans and ideas aside. Remind me of all that You have taught me in the difficult moments and seasons in my life so I will never forget how You kept your promises, defeated my doubt, and restored the things that were fractured within me.

"Remind me, God, that You knew me before you placed me here on Earth and that You love me still. Remind me that I am only visiting this world to glorify You. Remind me that You have determined the end of all things at the beginning and that nothing is a surprise to You. Remind me that everything that happens has been ordained by You . . . that I need not worry or fear the outcome for me and the ones I love, because You love them too; we are all a part of Your divine plan.§ Thank you, God, for defeating my disappointment, fears, and anxiety with Your presence. Thank you, Lord, for tethering me to Your goodness, Your grace, Your love, Your power, Your mercy, and Your strength. I pray that as I strive to be a better representative of You, my Lord, that my actions and thoughts will reflect my trust in You and that my actions and thoughts will reflect my gratitude for Your sacrifice and will honor Your magnificence."

I hope my experience will prevent you or someone you love from falling into the shrouded prison of pain, depression, and a substance or opioid use disorder. Do not believe the deceit of chronic pain—it is only a shadow. Put on courage and reach for support. Do no stop pursuing a fulfilled life or allow chronic pain to steal your hope for a future. Protect your hope so you can stand firmly on the reliable faithfulness of God.

> May the God of hope fill you with all joy and peace as you trust in Him, so that you may overflow with hope by the power of the Holy Spirit (Romans 15:13 NIV).

---

§ Psalms 139:16 . . . all the days ordained for me were written in your book before one of them came to be.

Endnotes

1. Dydyk A.M., Conermann T., *Chronic Pain*. [Updated 2022 Nov 7]. In: StatPearls [Internet]. Treasure Island (FL): StatPearls Publishing; 2023 Jan–. Available from: https://www.ncbi.nlm.nih.gov/books/NBK553030/

2. U.S. Census Bureau. https://www.census.gov/quickfacts/fact/table/US/POP010220

3. T.B. Crouch, S. Wedin, R.L. Kilpatrick, L. Christon, W. Balliet, J. Borckardt, and K. Barth, Medical University of South Carolina. 2020 American Psychological Association. *Pain Rehabilitation's Dual Power: Treatment for Chronic Pain and Prevention of Opioid-Related Risks.* https://www.apa.org/pubs/journals/releases/amp-amp0000663.pdf

4. Breivik H, Collett B, Ventafridda V, Cohen R, Gallacher D. *Survey of chronic pain in Europe: prevalence, impact on daily life, and treatment.* Eur J Pain. 2006 May;10(4):287-333. doi: 10.1016/j.ejpain.2005.06.009. Epub 2005 Aug 10. PMID: 16095934. https://pubmed.ncbi.nlm.nih.gov/16095934/

5. Raffaeli W, Arnaudo E. *Pain as a disease: an overview.* J Pain Res. 2017 Aug 21;10:2003–2008. doi: 10.2147/JPR.S138864. PMID:

28860855; PMCID: PMC5573040. https://www.ncbi.nlm.nih.gov /pmc/articles/PMC5573040/

6. https://www.nih.gov/news-events/news-releases/nih-study-finds -high-rates-persistent-chronic-pain-among-us-adults

7. Raffaeli W, Arnaudo E. *Pain as a disease: an overview.* J Pain Res. 2017 Aug 21;10:2003-2008. doi: 10.2147/JPR.S138864. PMID: 28860855; PMCID: PMC5573040. https://www.ncbi.nlm.nih.gov /pmc/articles/PMC5573040/

8. Mills SEE, Nicolson KP, Smith BH. *Chronic pain: a review of its epidemiology and associated factors in population-based studies.* Br J Anaesth. 2019 Aug;123(2):e273-e283. doi: 10.1016/j.bja.2019.03.023. Epub 2019 May 10. PMID: 31079836; PMCID: PMC6676152 https://www .ncbi.nlm.nih.gov/pmc/articles/PMC6676152/

9. Raffaeli W, Arnaudo E. *Pain as a disease: an overview.* J Pain Res. 2017 Aug 21;10:2003-2008. doi: 10.2147/JPR.S138864. PMID: 28860855; PMCID: PMC5573040. https://www.ncbi.nlm.nih.gov /pmc/articles/PMC5573040/

10. Philip A. Pizzo, M.D., and Noreen M. Clark, Ph.D. *Alleviating Suffering 101—Pain Relief in the United States,* https://www.nejm .org/doi/full/10.1056/NEJMp1109084

11. National Center for Health Statistics, National Vital Statistics System, mortality data file. https://www.cdc.gov/nchs/fastats/leading-causes-of -death.htm

12. Buchbinder, Rachelle Buchbinder, Rachelle et al. *Low back pain: a call for action*: The Lancet, Volume 391, Issue 10137, 2384—2388. https://www. thelancet.com/journals/lancet/article/PIIS0140-6736(18)30488-4/fulltext

13. https://spinehealth.org/article/spine-anatomy/

14. https://www.dea.gov/drug-information/drug-scheduling

15. https://www.deadiversion.usdoj.gov/drug_chem_info/gabapentin.pdf

16. https://www.pharmacytimes.com/view/gabapentin-presents-high -potential-for-misuse

17. https://nida.nih.gov/research-topics/addiction-science/words-matter -preferred-language-talking-about-addiction

18. Dydyk AM, Jain NK, Gupta M. Opioid Use Disorder: Evaluation and Management. 2024 Jan 17. In: StatPearls [Internet]. Treasure Island (FL): StatPearls Publishing; 2025 Jan–. PMID: 31985959. https://www.ncbi.nlm.nih.gov/books/NBK553166/

19. Dydyk AM, Jain NK, Gupta M. Opioid Use Disorder: Evaluation and Management. 2024 Jan 17. In: StatPearls [Internet]. Treasure Island (FL): StatPearls Publishing; 2025 Jan–. PMID: 31985959. https://www.ncbi.nlm.nih.gov/books/NBK553166/

20. Campbell LS, Coomer TN, Jacob GK, Lenz RJ. Gabapentin controlled substance status. J Am Pharm Assoc. https://pubmed.ncbi. nlm.nih.gov/33674205/

21. Dfarhud D, Malmir M, Khanahmadi M. Happiness & Health: The Biological Factors—Systematic Review Article. Iran J Public Health. 2014 Nov.;43(11):1468-77. PMID; PMCID: PMC4449495. https:// pubmed.ncbi.nlm.nih.gov/26060713/

22. Raffaeli W, Arnaudo E. *Pain as a disease: an overview.* J Pain Res. 2017 Aug 21;10:2003-2008. doi: 10.2147/JPR.S138864. PMID: 28860855; PMCID: PMC5573040. https://www.ncbi.nlm.nih.gov /pmc/articles/PMC5573040/

23. *The Voice of the Patient A series of reports from the U.S. Food and Drug Administration's (FDA's) Patient-Focused Drug Development Initiative* Chronic Pain Public Meeting: July 9, 2018 Report Date: March 2019. https://www.fda.gov/media/124390/download

24. *The Voice of the Patient A series of reports from the U.S. Food and Drug Administration's (FDA's) Patient-Focused Drug Development Initiative* Chronic Pain Public Meeting: July 9, 2018 Report Date: March 2019. https://www.fda.gov/media/124390/download

25. Szalavitz M, Rigg KK, Wakeman SE. *Drug dependence is not addiction—and it matters.* Ann Med. 2021 Dec;53(1):1989-1992. doi: 10.1080/07853890.2021.1995623. PMID: 34751058; PMCID: PMC8583742. https://www.ncbi.nlm.nih.gov/pmc/articles/PMC858 3742/

26. *The Voice of the Patient A series of reports from the U.S. Food and Drug Administration's (FDA's) Patient-Focused Drug Development Initiative* Chronic Pain Public Meeting: July 9, 2018 Report Date: March 2019. https://www.fda.gov/media/124390/download

27. American Psychiatric Association. *Diagnostic and statistical manual of mental disorders.* 5th ed, American Psychiatric Publishing, 2013. https://psycnet.apa.org/record/2013-14907-000

28. Nora D. Volkow, M.D. and A. Thomas McLellan, Ph.D. *Opioid Abuse in Chronic Pain—Misconceptions and Mitigation Strategies.* March 31, 2016. N Engl J Med 2016; 374:1253-1263 https://www .nejm.org/doi/full/10.1056/nejmra1507771

29. Psychogenic Pain. https://my.clevelandclinic.org/health/diseases/12056 -pain-psychogenic-pain

30. Nora D. Volkow, M.D. and A. Thomas McLellan, Ph.D. *Opioid Abuse in Chronic Pain—Misconceptions and Mitigation Strategies.* March 31, 2016. N Engl J Med 2016; 374:1253-1263 https://www .nejm.org/doi/full/10.1056/nejmra1507771

31. Nora D. Volkow, M.D. and A. Thomas McLellan, Ph.D. *Opioid Abuse in Chronic Pain—Misconceptions and Mitigation Strategies.*

March 31, 2016. N Engl J Med 2016; 374:1253-1263 https://www
.nejm.org/doi/full/10.1056/nejmra1507771

32. Drug Involved Overdose Deaths. https://nida.nih.gov/sites/default/files
/drug-involved-overdose-deaths-1999-2022.pptx

33. Drug Involved Overdose Deaths. https://nida.nih.gov/sites/default/files
/drug-involved-overdose-deaths-1999-2022.pptx

34. Raffaeli W, Arnaudo E. *Pain as a disease: an overview.* J Pain Res. 2017
Aug 21;10:2003-2008. doi: 10.2147/JPR.S138864. PMID: 28860855;
PMCID: PMC5573040. https://www.ncbi.nlm.nih.gov/pmc
/articles/PMC5573040/

35. Dydyk A.M., Conermann T., *Chronic Pain.* [Updated 2022 Nov 7].
In: StatPearls [Internet]. Treasure Island (FL): StatPearls Publishing;
2023 Jan–. Available from: https://www.ncbi.nlm.nih.gov/books
/NBK553030/

36. Ray BM, Kelleran KJ, Fodero JG, Harvell-Bowman LA. *Examining
the Relationship Between Chronic Pain and Mortality in U.S. Adults.*
J Pain. 2024 Oct;25(10):104620. doi: 10.1016/j.jpain.2024.104620.
Epub 2024 Jun 26. PMID: 38942415. Examining the Relationship
Between Chronic Pain and Mortality in U.S. Adults—PubMed.
https://pubmed.ncbi.nlm.nih.gov/38942415/

37. Jane C. Ballantyne, Mark D. Sullivan, *Is Chronic Pain a Disease?* The
Journal of Pain, Volume 23, Issue 10, 2022, Pages 1651-1665, ISSN
1526-5900. https://doi.org/10.1016/j.jpain.2022.05.001. https://www
.sciencedirect.com/science/article/pii/S1526590022003182

38. Ray BM, Kelleran KJ, Fodero JG, Harvell-Bowman LA. *Examining
the Relationship Between Chronic Pain and Mortality in U.S. Adults.*
J Pain. 2024 Oct;25(10):104620. doi: 10.1016/j.jpain.2024.104620.
Epub 2024 Jun 26. PMID: 38942415. Examining the Relationship

Between Chronic Pain and Mortality in U.S. Adults—PubMed. https://pubmed.ncbi.nlm.nih.gov/38942415/

39. https://my.clevelandclinic.org/health/diseases/16652-drug-addiction -substance-use-disorder-sud

40. Nora D. Volkow, M.D. and A. Thomas McLellan, Ph.D. *Opioid Abuse in Chronic Pain—Misconceptions and Mitigation Strategies.* March 31, 2016. N Engl J Med 2016; 374:1253-1263 https://www .nejm.org/doi/full/10.1056/nejmra1507771

41. Read H, Zagorac S, Neumann N, Kramer I, Walker L, Thomas E. Occupational Therapy: A Potential Solution to the Behavioral Health Workforce Shortage. Psychiatr Serv. 2024 Jul 1;75(7):703-705. https://psychiatryonline.org/doi/10.1176/appi.ps.20230298

42. https://www.who.int/news-room/fact-sheets/detail/musculoskeletal -conditions

43. Raffaeli W, Arnaudo E. *Pain as a disease: an overview.* J Pain Res. 2017 Aug 21;10:2003-2008. doi: 10.2147/JPR.S138864. PMID: 28860855; PMCID: PMC5573040. https://www.ncbi.nlm.nih.gov /pmc/articles/PMC5573040/

44. Dydyk A.M., Conermann T., *Chronic Pain.* [Updated 2022 Nov 7]. In: StatPearls [Internet]. Treasure Island (FL): StatPearls Publishing; 2023 Jan–. Available from: https://www.ncbi.nlm.nih.gov/books /NBK553030/

45. Meda RT, Nuguru SP, Rachakonda S, Sripathi S, Khan MI, Patel N. *Chronic Pain-Induced Depression: A Review of Prevalence and Management.* Cureus. 2022 Aug 25;14(8):e28416. doi: 10.7759/cureus.28416. PMID: 36171845; PMCID: PMC9509520. https://pubmed .ncbi.nlm.nih.gov/36171845/

46. https://www.who.int/news-room/fact-sheets/detail/musculoskeletal -conditions

References

Scriptures marked NIV are taken from the New International Version, Copyright 1973, 1978, 1984, 2011 by Biblica, Inc. https://you version.com/the-bible-app/

Scriptures marked NKJV are taken from the New King James Version, Copyright 1982 Thomas Nelson

https://www.youversion.com/the-bible-app/

Scriptures marked AMP are taken from the Amplified Bible, Copyright 2015 The Lockman Foundation https://www.youversion.com /the-bible-app/

Scriptures marked KJV are taken from the King James Version, in the United Kingdom, patentee Cambridge University Press

https://www.youversion.com/the-bible-app/ YouVersion (Version 10.15.1, RED 3.9.11.8182) {Mobile app}.

www.ingramcontent.com/pod-product-compliance
Lightning Source LLC
Chambersburg PA
CBHW070919130626
46555CB00001B/204